2nd EDITION

ASTON® POSTURAL ASSESSMENT

A New Paradigm for Evaluating Body Patterns

2nd EDITION

ASTON® POSTURAL ASSESSMENT

A New Paradigm for Evaluating Body Patterns

Judith Aston

Forewords

Thomas W Myers · Darlene Hertling

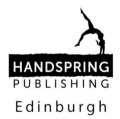

HANDSPRING PUBLISHING

Edinburgh

HANDSPRING PUBLISHING LIMITED
The Old Manse, Fountainhall,
Pencaitland, East Lothian
EH34 5EY, Scotland
Tel: +44 1875 341 859
Website: www.handspringpublishing.com

First edition published 1999 by Psychological Corp
Second edition published 2019 in the United Kingdom by Handspring Publishing

ISBN 978-912085-34-7
ISBN (Kindle eBook) 978-912085-35-4

British Library Cataloguing in Publication Data
A catalogue record for this book is available from the British Library
Library of Congress Cataloguing in Publication Data
A catalog record for this book is available from the Library of Congress

Notice
Neither the Publisher nor the Authors assume any responsibility for any loss or injury and/or damage to persons or property arising out of or relating to any use of the material contained in this book. It is the responsibility of the treating practitioner, relying on independent expertise and knowledge of the patient, to determine the best treatment and method of application for the patient.
All reasonable efforts have been made to obtain copyright clearance for illustrations in the book for which the author or publishers do not own the rights. If you believe that one of your illustrations has been used without such clearance please contact the publishers and we will ensure that appropriate credit is given in the next reprint.

Commissioning Editor Mary Law
Project Manager Morven Dean
Copy editor Susan Stuart
Cover designer Bruce Hogarth
Indexer Aptara, India
Typesetter Amnet Systems
Printer Replika Press, India

The
Publisher's
policy is to use
paper manufactured
from sustainable forests

CONTENTS

DEDICATION

I dedicate this book to the memory of the late Dr. Ida Rolf, who introduced me to her world of bodywork, fascia and transformation, and to all the practitioners who trained with her in the 1960s and 1970s, for their contributions to expanding the knowledge of her work around the world. Those practitioners' names will be listed on our website, at AstonKinetics.com.

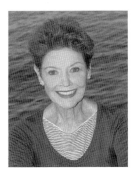

Judith Aston has had a lifelong interest in human movement and structure that has been informed by her studies of dance, psychology, and bodywork. She earned her BA and MFA from the University of California at Los Angeles, as well as a Lifetime Teaching Credential in Dance and Physical Education. Aston's experience in designing and teaching movement programs for Long Beach Community College and human potential workshops caught the attention of the renowned Dr. Ida Rolf, founder and developer of the connective system of body rehabilitation known as Structural Integration ('Rolfing'). At Aston's first session with Dr. Rolf in Big Sur, California, in April 1968, Dr. Rolf asked her to design a movement component for the Rolfing series, as a way for clients to sustain the effects of bodywork through self-awareness and movement re-education. Over the next nine years, Aston progressively developed the program called Structural Patterning, which she taught to all Structural Integration practitioner trainees and to those chosen to become movement instructors for the work.

This intensive exposure to many body patterns stimulated Aston's continual quest to understand optimal human alignment, structure and movement, in the field of gravity. As the practitioners learned, through Structural Patterning, to use their bodies more cooperatively and with less effort, Aston realized that the results visible in their clients' alignment and structural dimension seemed to differ from the standard plumb line alignment and the Rolf line.

By 1977, Aston understood that, in order to respect the integrity of both the Structural Integration system and her own developing perspective, she needed independence. Once the move was made, Aston's inexhaustible insights found form in creating specific trainings on Aston Fascial Integration (three myofascial forms of work, including the Aston massage, Arthro-Kinetics and Myo-Kinetics), six different forms of Aston® Fitness, as well as specific Aston® trainings for yoga, pilates, senior fitness, facial fitness, and athletes (runners, cyclists, swimmers, etc.).

Her emerging paradigm brought an opportunity to design products that matched her ideas of better ergonomics, which are offered through her office and website. All the specific courses are based on the unifying principles of the Aston® Paradigm, a new vision of human postural assessment and function. Today, in addition to lecturing and conducting classes on Aston® Kinetics in the United States, Europe and Australia, as well as on-line coaching, Aston designs ergonomic products for work, sports and home use, and is listed in the official *Who's Who of American Inventors*.

Judith is widely recognized as a visionary and pioneer in the art and science of kinetics, for her creation of the Aston Paradigm and its forms of honoring the individual's unique and changing body patterns. Her creativity abounds, with the development of Aston Kinetics and the creation of more than 200 formal training days of different content for Aston Kinetics. Aston offers classes on her educational systems for movement and bodywork near her home at Lake Tahoe, Nevada and at other locations. You can find more information about courses and schedules as well as blogs and videos on her website: AstonKinetics.com. This is her third book.

ACKNOWLEDGMENTS

It has been fun to add 21 more years of experience to the knowledge base of content for this book, the second edition. I have now been teaching for 56 years (starting at a college in 1963). I appreciate the questions and the need to problem-solve the body concerns that students, clients and teachers have presented to me. Thank you.

I want to thank all the students and clients who posed for photos: as for the earlier book (1998) we asked them to exaggerate their body postures to make it easier for readers to identify the specific patterns.

My team deserves much appreciation and acknowledgment for their many skills, talents, commitment and endurance. They are: **Maureen Mika** – not only is she our editor but she also took on the tasks of redoing all of the illustrations and editing photos from the first edition of this book, all of which involves many different skills and tremendous attention to detail, layout and design; **Weston Fettgather** took more than 350 new photos, in several photo shoots, and has spent many hours editing them. I also want to thank **Courtney Pennacchio**, who helped with transcribing, and cut and pasted numerous photos in the text with me, for specific demonstrations of a concept.

Thank you to **Ann Todhunter Brode**, a practitioner since the early 1970s, for her input and encouragement, **Ronnie Oliver**, advanced faculty, who has shared her abundant skills and perspectives for 45 years, and **Allison Sagewind**, advanced faculty, for her feedback, enthusiasm and generous support for the last 25+ years.

I wish to express my appreciation for all the people at Handspring and the freelance artists who added their talents, ideas, and support to make this book project materialize. They are Mary Law, Andrew Stevenson, Bruce Hogarth, Morven Dean, Susan Stuart, Hilary Brown, Martin Hill, Stephanie Ricks and Dylan Hamilton.

And finally, to my husband, **Brian Linderoth**, also an advanced faculty, for his incredible support, wisdom of the work, and his generosity that feels as though it comes from lifetimes of experience.

I have been fascinated by the ways people move and express themselves for as long as I can remember. I explored this passion by studying dance for many years; getting a degree in Physical Education; and teaching actors and athletes how their habitual patterns of moving could be changed to optimize their performance. In the 1960s, I pursued this absorbing interest to the Esalen Institute, where I collaborated with a Gestalt therapist to enable those attending to explore how movement, or lack thereof, reflects our inner lives.

Then, in 1968, after several years of intractable pain resulting from auto accidents, a friend encouraged me to meet with Dr. Ida Rolf, who was seeing patients at Esalen and teaching her system of bodywork, Structural Integration ('Rolfing'). Her work introduced into our popular culture the idea that bodies can change as a result of very specific 'hands-on' bodywork, and that we are not condemned to slowly become more and more debilitated from accidents and the effects of age. Dr. Rolf had heard of my own work and invited me to develop a series of movement exercises based on her model, which we called 'Rolf-Aston Structural Patterning', in order to allow students to sustain the results of their bodywork sessions.

I worked with Dr. Rolf and taught her students for nine illuminating years, during which I was constantly modifying the program based on my observations, in order to make it more effective. One of the most surprising results that the practitioners began to notice was that, when they learned how to use their bodies in this new way, their work became less effortful and created less discomfort in their clients.

Over time, I saw that my insights had actually developed into a new paradigm, an evolution from previous thought about human alignment and movement. Today, this paradigm underlies all forms of Aston® Kinetics movement education and bodywork: Aston® Massage, Myo-Kinetics, Arthro-Kinetics, Aston® Fitness, and ergonomic products and applications.

In this book I share some of the underlying perspectives and rationale for the basic principles of the Aston® Paradigm, developed through my 56 years of teaching. I've also included exercises to help the reader progressively train their own seeing and evaluation skills because I believe that we need to learn to see 'what is' in order to know where we need to go.

These parameters for postural assessment can be integrated into any practice concerned with optimizing human well-being, everyday movement, or specialized performance. Students have reported that learning these skill-sets has changed their practice significantly, enabling them to achieve more lasting benefits more quickly and with less effort.

I hope this is true for you as well.

Judith Aston

FOREWORD by Thomas W Myers

Finally, and hooray! Judith Aston has laid out her philosophy, vision, and a thorough tour of her assessment method in one big book. This is a cause for celebration, followed by the necessity to sit down quietly, take up this material, and apply it practically to your clients or students.

That is not so hard – the book in your hand is the most comprehensive book about postural analysis you are likely to find in this lifetime, as it synthesizes decades of close observation and extensive multi-modal practice. Judith's material is also laid out in a logical manner to facilitate assimilation and progressive practice.

Somatotyping and visual assessment are both an art and a craft, and not so much a science – not yet. The first task is to master the basics of the craft of seeing. From there on in, insight – the ability to 'see in' – is a progressive love affair like every art. Judith's methodology in this book is a very real 'leg up' to the craft. Go watch her in action to appreciate her marriage of practical craft with the art of moving through life.

From the outset, however, I recommend that you clarify the distinction in your mind between 'function' – doing – and 'posture', which is more about where you *are* – being. Posture is where you start from, your postural pattern says more about who you are than what you do.

Of course, the two are related – what you do shapes how you stand, and how you are limits or facilitates what functions you can perform. As Wainwright put it: 'Structure without Function is a corpse; Function without Structure is a ghost.' Yet it is very much worth the work of discerning the distinction between the two.

Much of the emphasis in contemporary rehabilitation and athletic or artistic performance enhancement is on what tasks you can and cannot *do*. Recently, varying approaches claim the label 'functional', with popular screening tests that measure range of motion, strength, and core abilities. All well and good. Now that those basic competencies are laid out, let us ask: Where are you starting from? As did, in their different ways, both Drs Ida Rolf and Moshe Feldenkrais: Where are you 'at home' in your body? To make it more complicated, most of us have a number of postures: sitting, sleeping, walking, working, moving along scales of alert/fatigued, empowered/burdened, introvert/extrovert, etc.

Judith Aston's comprehensive approach simplifies the work – but simple does not mean easy. Allow yourself to fumble through your first 50 attempts at this kind of body reading in your practice before you give up on yourself or this method. Recognizing relationships takes looking closely and just puzzling it out on at least a few dozen people before the patterns begin to reveal themselves and you start working in relationships, not working 'on' something. Then you will be off to the races on your own lifetime's worth of hunting in the wilderness of human movement patterns. Judith offers you a simple set of steps, one after the other, building to greater and greater skill.

An example of structural/functional mismatch: most right-handed weekend-warrior tennis players have the right shoulder lower than the left, as the right side draws in and down via the lat, abs, serratus, and quadrates lumborum. These amateur players often 'punch' at the ball from the shoulder (which leads to valgus strain down the medial inter muscular septum – 'tennis elbow' – and in they come to your practice).

This is not ideal: most professional tennis players learn to rotate through their medial axis, around the spine, which uses both right and left side nearly equally, despite the racquet always being in their right hand. It is difficult to get there, but once achieved, the player gains more grace, power, and stamina. Nevertheless, most less than divinely gifted players go through a period of powering the ball with a lowered right shoulder. Go see. (All this is left for the southpaw player.)

xiv

Now, if someone takes up tennis who happens to have their left shoulder lower than their right – due to whatever accident, dominant eye, genetics, or other cause – they are not likely to thrive at tennis and may soon give it up: 'I'm not good at this.' Or, if they like it too much to give it up, they are likely to shift their posture toward the right shoulder being in the advantageous 'down' position, which is usually not a 'corrective', but simply piles more tension onto the posture they had before.

Everybody who comes to you is a complicated pattern of 'being' and 'doing' woven with each other over myriad decisions, accidents, surgeries, loves won and lost, aversions, and predispositions. It is the practitioner's job to unravel – 'unwind' as it is now called – these patterns back to something like 'natural', untrammelled movement – and then they will have an easier time relaxing into length and centering their swing around the central axis.

Everything in here has daily value, and the art of postural assessment deepens over time with practice, following the stairs step-by-step up 'the leaning tower of Pisa' of the various odd and inefficient patterns people manage to put themselves into – through imitation, injury, and attitude – all mediated by the shadowless force of gravity working on our 70,000,000,000,000 cells and their fascial matrix. Judith gives you strings to follow out of the labyrinth of postural confusion (and it can be confusing) into the light of understanding that leads to 'Here is what I am going to do next.'

I personally could not be more grateful to Judith Aston. I, too, was drawn into the orbit of Dr. Ida Rolf in the 1970s, a few years after Judith, but in those halcyon days when she was still teaching with Rolf's institute. My contact with her was glancing – a couple of four-day classes and a few sessions in those early days – but she has had a profound effect on my practice for over 40 years since then.

It has been my privilege to take further training, and to sponsor her to teach for my students in the Anatomy

Trains School, so I have had additional contact with her skill-set over the years. The deep effect of those initial days in class and the sessions that accompanied them have been a source of learning in my practice over many, many years.

Not only my practice: for one memorable session I took my guitar with me, and she gave me a lesson about where I came from when I sang and played. It was hard at first – habit is a strong enemy, tough to break – but by working with my pelvic position suddenly the guitar felt light, my breath deepened, and everyone watching the session (it was in a class she was teaching) heard the difference when I performed from this new place. I have never gone back.

Oops, not true. I do go back. When I am tired or out of sorts, I do find myself hunched over the guitar, singing in a tight, 1960's Dylanesque voice. But the discomfort and the choke on my musical expression is immediately evident to me and I correct into the easier support and more open tone. 'Judith,' I said to her some years later, 'You've ruined my slump.' This was my opened door to a more mindful relating to others in a variety of circumstances.

Judith's work is profound, and her consummate ability is to imitate the movement of others then break it down into its component pieces, so you can also see it and put it together. I will never be as good as she is at it, but much of the insight in the Anatomy Trains 'BodyReading®' derives from the insight into posture I was fortunate to receive at the knees of Ida Rolf and Judith Aston.

'Mindfulness' is a buzzword these days, and the first thing we need to be mindful of is our bodies: its sensations, feelings, hunches, hidden pains, lost places, restrictions, and joys. A large part of how we assemble our moment-by-moment perception rests on the sensations formed through our kinaesthetic sense. Judith is a master of bringing mindfulness to bear on the pattern of movement in the body.

Prepare for a feast. Know that this meal will keep nourishing you long after you have first tasted its joys. With a bit of investment – practice, practice, practice these skills – you will become a cook, linking your practice, whatever it is, to your assessment of posture, of where your client is coming from. I cannot emphasize enough how this will help you get them where you (and they) want to go.

Thomas W Myers
Director, Anatomy Trains
Maine, USA
July 2019

FOREWORD by Darlene Hertling

In these analyses of postural alignment and muscle balance, Judith Aston presents the first part of her published work on Aston® Kinetics, which is her own creation. This excellent book, originally a synthesis of the author's unique teaching courses, has now matured into a very practical text, a triumph of orderly thought and presentation. This study presents only one aspect of Aston Kinetics, which is an integrated system of movement education, three-dimensional soft tissue work, fitness training, and ergonomics. It is unique among the somatic disciplines in its completeness. Aston Kinetics includes a comprehensive formal evaluative system, innovative manual techniques that are applicable to a wide range of dysfunction in the musculoskeletal system, a number of exercise programs designed to develop a particular aspect of fitness, movement education procedures, and an array of fundamental concepts that allow the work to have an extraordinary scope of application.

Aston Kinetics presents a system of therapy that has grown out of creative observation and consistent, independent development. One that, in its manner of observing and interpreting human movement and alignment, I have long regarded as a fundamental contribution to the field of a variety of therapies. Although no explicit references are cited, this work accords with the findings of modern neuro-physiology and biomechanics in every field. The preventative and therapeutic value of more optimal posture and movement, and the conception of the human being as an organism constantly reacting with gravity, ground reaction force, and other external stimuli, are inherent in this system.

The major focus of this text is viewing static posture and alignment containing a series of exercises for learning, in order for the therapist to facilitate a greater appreciation of the structure of the human body. The thoroughness of presentation gives the therapist immediate access to meaningful, practical work and will allow them to form a basis from which to extend their knowledge of human structure to economical movement therapy: *seeing* structurally, from the aspect of alignment, dimension, and proportion. Alignment deals with the placement of the body and its parts. The relationship of parts in space and the distribution of weight-bearing through these parts are two aspects of alignment. Dimension and proportion concern the internal volume of the body or a body part, and how that volume is distributed with regard to its component dimensions of width, length and depth. The three-dimensional position in space of each skeletal part can also be determined. Deviations from normal are expressed in biomechanical terms such as rotation, shear, and compression.

Another component of Aston Kinetics is the correlation of alignment patterns to muscle tone. In assessing muscle tension, the examiner observes and palpates the tension patterns throughout the body and notates areas where there is excessive or lack of tension that might be inappropriate. This body map creates a visual record of the body's patterns.

The level of integration between bodywork, movement education, and ergonomics, as well as the recognition of asymmetry in structure and movement, and the individual problem-solving for each patient are unique to this approach. This text introduces Aston seeing skills as a basis for evaluating posture. The thoroughness in presentation of this work gives the therapist immediate access to meaningful, practical work and will enable them to develop an unlimited and eminently individualized program of patient care.

It should be remembered that what we see is profoundly influenced by the way we look. Every individual tends to take the limits of their own perception also to be the limits of the perceived world, and a cardinal error is to see clinical problems only in one's own idiom. A healthy eclectic approach offsets this otherwise limited trend.

Darlene Hertling, PT
Senior Lecturer Emerita,
Department of Rehabilitation Medicine
University of Washington, Seattle
Washington, USA
June 2019

My intention for this book is two-fold: 1) To clearly show how the traditional way of evaluating the dysfunction and ideal structure of our bodies needs to be revised in order to move toward our full potential, and 2) to provide a step-by-step manual for practitioners to learn this evolutionary way of seeing and to include these insights in their own practices. Students often ask me 'How did you come up with this?' and I hope that, by including some of my personal experiences and empirical observations, I will be able to illustrate how the Aston® Paradigm evolved into the foundation for all of the Aston® Kinetics modalities.

This book focuses on the first essential skills taught in the Aston® Work curriculum, 'Seeing the Body: Postural Assessment'. In Chapter 8, I have shared some of the underlying perspectives and rationale for the basic principles of the Aston® Paradigm, as well as exercises to help the reader progressively train their own seeing and evaluation skills. I explain why the observational plumb line needs to shift forward from its traditional location in order to allow for the natural dimensional integrity of the body to appear. I believe that we also need to appreciate how our bodies have a natural functional asymmetry that reflects our physiology and allows us to enter into movement, rather than projecting an unreasonable expectation of symmetry onto a dynamic system.

Just as any movement can be broken down into its component parts, assessment of the body's proportion, structure and functioning can be made by accurately reading each individual part, its relationship to another part, its relation to the whole structure, and, finally, its availability to the force of gravity and ground reaction force. We need to see 'what is' in the context of the theoretical 'neutral' in order to know where we need to go. From there we can evaluate the compromises that are being made in the optimal structure and function of the body and how the dimensions and alignment of each part interact.

Accurate assessment and clear notation allow the practitioner to track the changes from session to session and to deduce whether some essential element is being overlooked. They can also reveal what is more causal and what is more secondary in the client's patterns, which allows for a more efficient sequencing of session work. Application of these observational and analytical skills makes whatever techniques are used more effective.

Beginnings and influences

Something in my nature has always allowed me to see with great accuracy the ways bodies move, and has provided the empirical foundation for my work. My mother told me that, when I was as young as four, I somehow had the skill of being able to mime people's body patterns and motions so well that my family knew who I was imitating. I would say 'A lady came by with these papers for you.' 'What was her name?' 'I don't know but she walked like this...' My mother would laugh and say 'Oh, that's Mrs Brown!'

I would dance around the house constantly. My mother said that she enrolled me in the local dance studio as the only way to have some peace and quiet. I studied and performed recitals with this studio until I was 14.

For three years in high school I assisted Mrs Martha Walker in her classes for blind students. Her husband, Mr Del Walker, was the head of the Physical Education department at the college. In 1963, when I was 21, I was hired by Long Beach Community College to set up a Dance Department and to create and teach movement programs for the Physical Education, Theatre, Music and Community Education departments on their recommendation.

This funny story illustrates one of the experiences that influenced how I developed the Aston-Kinetics curricula so many years later. One of the classes I was required to teach the athletes was Social Dance. Whenever one of the students, a talented runner who had won many 440 m events, was trying to do the foxtrot, he awkwardly seemed to be weighted on one foot while trying to step on the same foot. When I asked his buddies if there was some concern I should know about, they said 'Are you kidding? Come to practice and see for yourself.' I watched him run: he was smooth, efficient and graceful. I had to determine what was getting in his way when he was asked to dance and how to interrupt that unsuccessful pattern of thought and movement. I intuitively tapped into the movements that his body was accustomed to: instead of teaching dance moves, I asked him to perform series of slow and fast runs, forward and backward and to either side. I held onto his hands while facing him and as I gradually led him into the foxtrot box step, he said 'Miss Aston, I'm dancing!' Coach Walker had been watching all of this, and when he caught up with me he remarked that I had an interesting running style. This was puzzling to me at the time, as I would jump, skip and run without any conception about how to do the actions. I learned later how to break down any movement pattern into its component actions, actions that could each be 're-patterned' through a combination of first releasing unnecessary tensions and then learning new, more efficient and less effortful, natural movement sequences. Even later, I discovered how to use the Earth's laws of gravity and ground reaction force to assist us as we move through our lives.

In 1964 I started my masters program at UCLA. I had taken introductions to both psychology and theatre. But somehow it became my focus to combine dance with theatre and psychology for my thesis. The relationship between movement and the psyche has continued to be a life-long interest, and one of the elements in the Aston-Kinetics training. I find that our bodies manifest their interpretations of emotion, fatigue, anxiety, enthusiasm, etc., and that all of these states have a corresponding influence on the body's chemistry and holding patterns, which need to be neutralized before they become our new normal.

I offered my first Stage Movement course in 1965. It quickly became apparent that the young acting students were limited in their character expression by their lack of awareness of their own body postures and habitual movement patterns. They needed to be able to see posture and movement in order to build character expressions that were clearly different from their own.

Around the same time I had been asked to create movement programs for a human potential center, Kairos, in La Jolla, California. These participants included group leaders from the Esalen Institute as well as many other experts in the fields of psychology, movement, bodywork and the human potential movement. One of the psychiatrists asked me if I could create a program for his patients who attended his weekend seminars at Kairos.

Then, in late 1966 and mid-1967 I had two serious car accidents. In one, I was rear-ended by someone going 50+ miles an hour when I was at a stop. This left me in a great deal of back and sciatic pain – I was unable to fully stand up, and I was slightly bent over with most of my weight over my right leg. At the conclusion of my course of physical therapy, I was shocked and angered when the final report from the hospital said that they could find no real cause for my pain and that it must be in my head. I consulted the psychiatrist from Kairos who had commissioned my work, saying that the pain felt physically real. He believed me, and recommended that I should see Dr Ida Rolf, who would be visiting Esalen in the spring of 1968.

When I arrived in Big Sur, California, Dr Rolf was fully booked with client sessions, and so I sat on her doorstep for two days until she had a cancellation and I had my first session. I knew immediately that she was someone who knew how to change body patterns and improve function. She must have made enquiries into who the strange woman was sitting on her doorstep, because at the end of my first session she said that she'd heard I created movement programs for people. When I said yes, she asked if I could create a movement program for her work, Structural Integration ('Rolfing'). I immediately said 'Yes!' I didn't think about the 'when' until she said, 'Well, I will have to train you and the class starts this June.' This was a surprise to me as no-one had ever needed to train me – when I'd been asked to consult or develop a movement program previously, I would observe the work or class as it was currently, come in with a few ideas to be applied, and then I'd evaluate the feedback. After that I would expand and finalize the program for the client. When I asked Dr Rolf why, she said, 'So you will know what to do'. I apologized to her, as I had plans to go to Europe and didn't think I could change them. To which Dr Rolf replied, 'The class starts in six weeks, change your plans.' That was the way Dr. Rolf was. I said 'OK' and that was that!

I studied and worked with Dr Rolf for nine years. During that time I created and taught many classes for her Structural Integration students – around 200 people. All the Structural Integration students were required to take my first four-day class on seeing body patterns and on efficient body mechanics. I also trained about 50 movement education teachers. This early movement work was called Rolf-Aston Structural Patterning.

I created this form to apply Dr Rolf's ideas about alignment and correct postures so that clients could sustain the changes brought about through their bodywork sessions. Because this early work was informed by Dr Rolf's paradigm, I used to teach people how to maintain their posture by using cues like, 'letting the top of the head go up'. I used these cues before I learned that the 'up' in the body can easily come from the ground.

By late 1975 I began to move with great speed to develop my own discoveries, and to train teachers, psychotherapists and bodyworkers in these new ideas that were coming to me, realizations that I could not ignore about posture, movement, fitness, and ergonomics. I could envision how these new ideas would change much about movement coaching, performance of exercise, sports, everyday activities and ergonomics. I developed a system that allowed practitioners to learn how to clearly analyze body structure and alignment.

And I was fascinated by the challenge of how to teach in a positive, effective way – how to assist the client to learn in a place based on the YES instead of what not to do, based on the NO. I'd begun this approach with that first college runner, and after 16 years of teaching, I could see the differences in the amount the student learned and retained. Learning on the 'yes' allows more information to come into one's awareness and use.

Over time, these insights developed into a new paradigm, an evolution from previous thought about human alignment and movement. Today this paradigm underlies all forms of Aston Kinetics movement education and bodywork (Aston Massage, Myo-Kinetics, Arthro-Kinetics), Aston Fitness, and ergonomic products and applications.

In my 55 years of teaching, I have had the opportunity to apply my discoveries and techniques to numerous applications, and the process always includes 'seeing': postural assessment. Seeing skills can help the Yoga and Pilates teacher, coach, fitness trainer, or physical therapist, to quickly identify a stressful body pattern and to use their skills to lessen the negative consequences of that pattern. This can result in providing relief of discomfort or the ability to change the biomechanics, enabling the client to improve their performance – to run faster, throw a ball with more power, recover from soccer practice more quickly, play a musical instrument with greater facility and expressiveness. I love helping people develop the skills to 'read' their own body so that they can evaluate for themselves what they need and what is helpful. This knowledge may feel 'subtle' at the beginning but, in time, it is possible to experience how specific modifications make real differences. People often want you to fix or correct a long list of complaints in their body. When we can see the whole-body pattern, we see how these isolated areas are connected. In fact, the isolated areas may be doing the best they can to negotiate the stresses placed upon them. When the therapist, teacher or coach can identify and work to neutralize the whole-body pattern, often the isolated areas of stress improve as well.

How is your eye? Can you spot when a painting on the wall is slightly off-center?

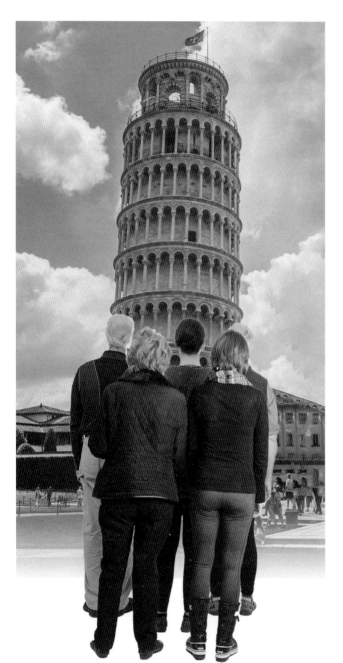

Have you ever been in a museum and noticed how some people looking at the art lean in the same direction as the subject they are looking at?

Do you find that sometimes you end up leaning to see the same perspective?

How about the Leaning Tower of Pisa? Can you tell it is about 6 degrees off-center?

What about these bodies? Are they off-center?

What are the consequences when the body is off its center?

It seems to be an accepted idea that the two sides of the body and face should be symmetrical – almost a mirror image of each other.

Now, let's look at this client together. At first glance, he looks fairly centered.

1) Maybe he has more weight on his left leg than his right leg.

2) Then maybe at his xyphoid (end of sternum), he looks like he shifts his chest a bit to the right.

3) You may notice his arm position, with his right hand facing in toward his body and his left hand facing back, more toward the wall behind him.

4) His hair looks like it stands up a bit more on his right side and his head may tend to tilt to his left.

Overall, nothing extreme, right?

If you take a string of dental floss and place it midway between his feet, perpendicular to the horizontal photo border, you can see where he balances most of his body weight. Which, in this case, is more to his left.

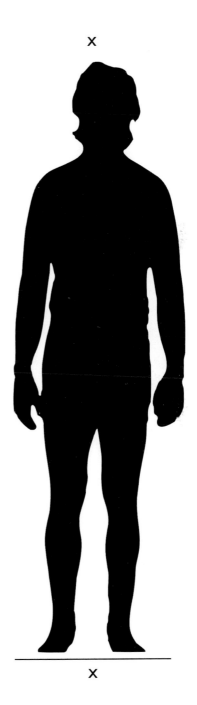

On the next page, compare how he might look with two right sides, and two left sides together.

x

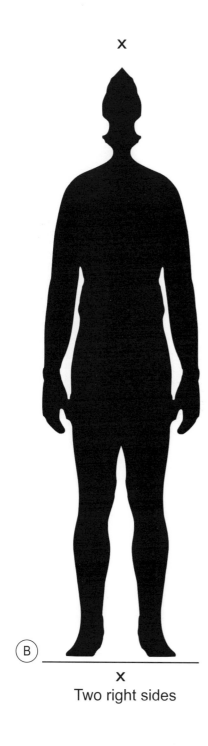

x

Two right sides

x

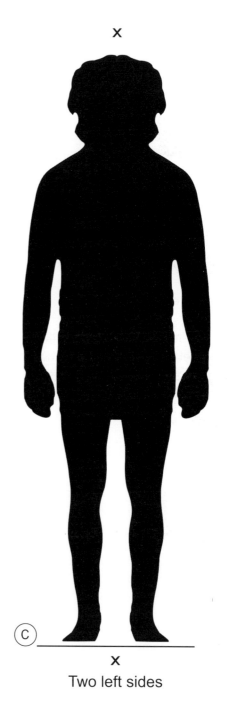

x

Two left sides

Now, compare all three perspectives together:

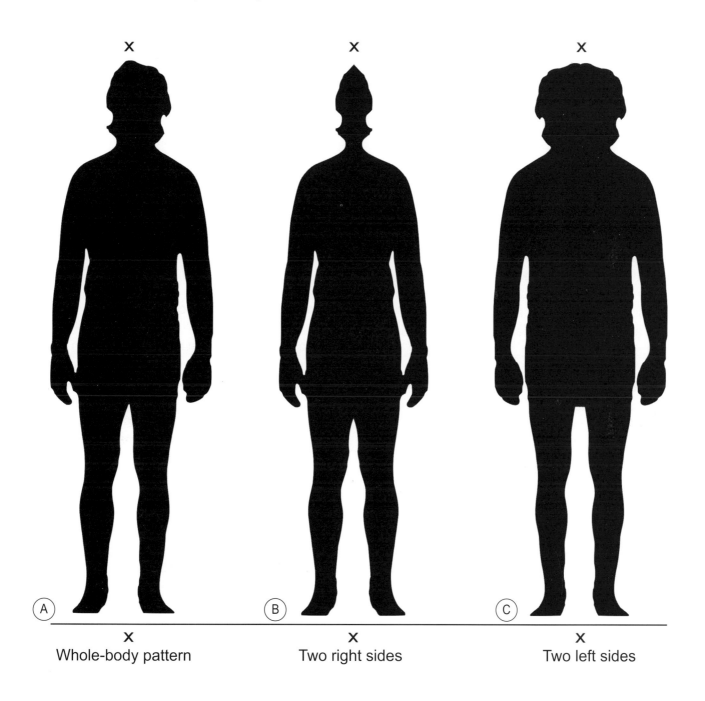

A	B	C
X	X	X
Whole-body pattern	Two right sides	Two left sides

It is surprising how different his two sides (B and C) look from this example. I hope this book will help train your eye to see the finer details of posture.

Introduction

Seeing posture

Movement instructors, manual therapists, dancers and coaches must learn how to see bodies. Some people see according to a (two-dimensional) grid, and that may work for their particular system, but being able to see the whole body, three-dimensionally, is most useful.

Alignment and posture

Alignment refers to the body's structure and how its parts are positioned to make up the whole. Understanding alignment includes knowing how a body is designed to work and how its design influences function. It also includes knowledge of the body's restrictions (such as a fused spine, a hip replacement, a scoliosis pattern) and what expectations or limitations those alignments would create. Alignment can be seen as more *structural*.

Posture is more about the body's usage. We can have good posture, bad posture and everything in between. Though we may have some of the alignment challenges mentioned above, we can probably still relax and slouch, or stand up with more tone and be in 'good posture'. Posture can reflect our mood, our energy level, recent surgeries, sensitivity to motion, and so on. Posture can be seen as more *functional*.

I mainly teach how to see the body and its patterns to manual therapists, coaches and those who teach movement disciplines. I use the term *postural assessment* to encompass the range from structural availability to habit, preference and usage.

When the body has specific restrictions, people often believe that they will never be any better. Not that therapists can replace missing bones, but often the skeleton is held in a certain position, without full range of motion, by soft tissue adhesions. When therapists tap into the body's innate ability to heal, and give the

right options for better movement, clients are surprised that what seemed so permanent is not. Alignment can change as soft tissues change, creating space and freedom for the skeleton to function more optimally. When body segments can fit their designated spaces better, the body in general and its organs specifically, can function better as well.

Educators and therapists are challenged daily with questions:

'Why am I getting tense here?'

'Why is this symptom occurring?'

'How could I have injured my neck while running?'

'Why don't I feel more balanced?'

'Why does my right side get overstressed during yoga, when my sister takes the same class and she doesn't get hurt?'

Numerous factors are to be considered when beginning to answer some of these questions. The content of this book focuses on body posture: the spatial position of the body segments in relationship to each other and to the whole body. We will also examine the possible consequences of posture on the body's shape. It is not the intent of this book to focus on the body's systems – cardiovascular, digestive, endocrine, respiratory, lymphatic, musculoskeletal, nervous, reproductive, and urinary. While it is obvious that the health of all the body's systems influence posture, I would like for you to consider how posture may influence all the body's systems.

As we, in the field, gain mastery of the skills that: 1) enable us to collect detailed and accurate information about our clients, and 2) apply it to help clients achieve and maintain optimal function, the better equipped we'll be to assist our clients to: 1) become his or her own teacher, and 2) know when and how to take charge of their own progress.

In this book, we will focus on the first skill, visual observation. However, there is another factor that many people in the therapeutic and coaching professions are beginning to see as a necessary component in their assessment. That is the ability to observe whole-body patterns.

Using specific testing to assess an individual body segment tells us everything about that segment in isolation. It reveals little, however, about the relationship of the particular segment to the whole body, and the possibility that the dysfunction of that segment is caused by its relationship to other body segments, through the forces of shear, compression, traction and rotation. For example, an ankle does not pronate independently of the knee or the pelvis above it; every exaggerated spinal curve has a significant effect on leg position and tension. It is these interrelationships that give us deeper insight when studying the whole body.

In practice, we commonly assess patients with multiple complaints, complex histories, and various structural changes in their bodies. People are interacting with the results of many years of habitual movement patterns and trauma, both physical and emotional. If we look at the interrelationships in the body, then an area of complaint may only be a starting place, a point of departure for assessment. By taking into consideration the functional relationships of the body, we can often trace the dysfunction from the site of complaint backward, to important underlying factors.

I have developed a great appreciation for the body's complexity over more than 50 years of teaching. I've taught thousands of therapists, teachers, coaches and athletes to analyze these relationships, in order to improve the results of their work. Learning to see from this perspective will introduce you to a different, and more dynamic, biomechanical paradigm for observing human structure and function.

Influences on posture

There are many influences on body structure and function. Interestingly, the chronological sequence of past events has, in conjunction with all other influences, determined our specific alignment (structure) and posture (function). For example, children commonly fall and hit their heads, badly bruise themselves, or break bones. A child is considered to be well when the bone mends, or the bruise or the headache is gone; however, the injury may have pushed a segment out of alignment, which the body then adapts to by counterbalancing. Therefore a single childhood injury event may set a postural pattern into motion, leaving one part of the body off-center to compensate for the area of injury. The child then grows up around the injury instead of growing through that area, inclusively. Subsequent injuries may then lay other compensations on top of the first, and so on.

Usually there is a reason that body parts align themselves as they do. The body shows an innate wisdom as it adopts alignment deviations or compensations in order to maintain its balance. Generally, bodies are very smart and do not make mistakes. They do the best they can to negotiate with their history, injuries, compensations, tasks and abilities to accomplish an action. However, often the body unconsciously holds on to these adaptive compensations long after they are needed. The result is an overall loss of full potential and freedom of movement.

I have found the body to be quite resilient in its ability to correct the adverse effects of compensating, given the appropriate formulas for neutralizing negative patterns. It is rewarding when, as therapists, teachers and coaches, we are able to facilitate change, neutralize a negative consequence, and help a person move and perform more optimally. It is important to remember that changing one body segment affects the whole system. By stepping back and looking at one part, in relation to the whole body, our view becomes more comprehensive and clear.

When we see the body as an integrated system rather than as many isolated segments, we recognize that we are a complete system, in stationary balance and in motion. Being able to see and understand this system greatly enhances our ability to facilitate change.

Take a moment to consider some of the influences that have shaped us:

1) Genetics
2) In-utero and birth experience
3) Developmental phases
4) Parental/caregiver patterns of holding, carrying, etc.
5) Product designs (e.g., furniture, tools, infant seats, shoes)
6) Appliances (e.g., braces, glasses, casts)
7) Role models (e.g., teachers, movie stars, athletes)
8) Fashions
9) Activities (e.g., baseball, swimming, golf, martial arts)
10) Current age, weight, state of health
11) Attitudes, beliefs, personality
12) Occupation (e.g., sedentary, lifting heavy equipment)
13) Nutrition, diet, addictions
14) Environment (e.g., community, altitude, pollution, noise)
15) Physics

Common assessment examples

In order for therapists, trainers, and coaches to assist someone in changing a pattern, it is necessary to be able to observe and assess that person's pattern as a starting point.

As a **physical therapist**: I might think I can see that the center of your trunk is placed posteriorly to the center of your pelvis (a compensation your body made during recovery from two broken legs) and that it left your balance precarious because your trunk is centered posteriorly to your foot at heel strike. If I can facilitate a more neutral alignment then I can help your gait pattern be more direct.

As a **massage therapist**: If I can quickly assess your overall body pattern in alignment, then I can correlate that information with what I feel in your musculoskeletal tissues and better design a session for overall improvement.

As a **personal trainer**: If I can see how your current alignment pattern contributes to your neck and shoulder tension when you lift a weight, then I can help you change that pattern throughout your whole body in order to avoid being overstressed.

As a **psychotherapist**: If I can see that your current alignment pattern no longer matches your current expression but is a flexed-ribcage posture that once matched feelings of grief, then I can form a strategy to help you.

As an **occupational therapist**: If I can see your body postural pattern, I can teach you whole-body usage for improving your ADLs (activities of daily living).

As an **ergonomics consultant**: If I can see your patterns of lumbar hyperextension and hyperflexion in your thoracic curve in relation to your being seated in a low chair all day, I can suggest changing your whole-body usage, to assist the isolated area of complaint (thoracic outlet), while sitting. I may also want to suggest a better chair design for you.

Introduction

Goals of this book

People often complain about an isolated area – lower back, shoulder, neck, knee, headaches – and so therapists are asked to work only on that one area. Many therapists trained in Aston seeing skills find it rewarding to be able to see, quickly and accurately, the interrelationships between the involved area and the contributing areas, and then be able to accelerate overall improvement while reducing the specific symptom.

People I have trained have consistently commented on three things about Aston seeing skills that are of particular value to them:

1) The Aston Paradigm provides a different perspective on neutral alignment.

2) Aston seeing skills help them understand how the dimensions of each body part interact with segmental alignment.

3) Most significantly, seeing skills help therapists attain an understanding of the interrelationships between body segments and their consequences.

Whether you are a novice or experienced therapist, teacher, coach or trainer, or a student in these arts, it is my hope that you will find this approach to be fresh, inspiring and of great practical use in your work.

This book has been created to provide a comprehensive self-teaching tool for developing **seeing skills**. These include:

1) Accurately assessing the segments of the body in three-dimensional space, including consideration of alignment and dimensions, or volume, of segments.

2) Understanding how these specific segmental interrelationships can create or secure hyper- and hypotonicity, and/or hyper- and hypomobility that perpetuate the body pattern.

This book also offers **tools**, to enable you to observe a client's body and quickly identify whole-body relationships that may contribute to an area of interest or complaint:

1) Experiences to develop and enhance observational skills.

2) Notation techniques, to assist easy visual recall for recording observations.

3) A process for summarizing your assessments, to create a plan for your client.

These elements of assessment are the precursors to therapeutic choices such as the work sequence, modalities, and areas of focus. However, detailed information on designing treatment plans based on your visual assessments is outside the scope of this book.

The Aston Paradigm has spawned a new perspective for evaluating musculoskeletal function – an evolution in movement education, fitness, product design, massage, and bodywork – and different ergonomic guidelines. It is because of the positive feedback I have received about the value of this information, from health care and fitness professionals who have been trained to use these techniques, that I have created this book.

Beyond the scope of this book is an entire system of movement education, bodywork and fitness programs that has grown from these ideas, as well as numerous product designs. Our website (AstonKinetics.com) includes many examples for your consideration and exploration.

How to use this book

The exercises and examples given in this book are designed to impart information and to develop skills in a specific sequence. This is a hands-on approach that will enable this two-dimensional medium to communicate more accurately the three-dimensional reality we are exploring. I encourage you to take the time to work through all the exercises.

Although you may have experience in analyzing alignment, this paradigm may use different landmarks – a different view of optimal alignment. Going through step by step will enable you to become familiar with this perspective.

The material is arranged from simple to complex relationships. Each section contains the repetition of a skill through a variety of examples. This is based on a learning model that suggests the information becomes more fully and easily integrated when one masters a skill before moving on to a new concept or skill. Therefore, certain pieces of information will be presented in isolated, two-dimensional or oversimplified forms at first. Each piece will be woven into the complex framework of the three-dimensional reality of the body by the conclusion.

Generally, each section includes text, examples and exercises for applying the ideas and some implications and clinical examples or applications. You may want to go through the book the first time just working with the development of skills. Then go through again and include the application of the concepts to practice. Others may find it most useful to see the implications for practice as they build skills. At any rate, you have the option to go through the entire text using just one of these tracks or combining them in any way you choose. Each way is a different experience and it may be useful at different times. In this way, the content expands as your experience increases and questions change. I have designed this book so that you may

write in it. The skill sets require practice so that you can use them with ease.

In the exercises, I have suggested that you make marks on the drawings and photos. (For those of you who prefer not to mark in your book, I suggest that you use tracing paper or transparencies and a dry-erase marker, to enable you to do the exercises, erase, and move on.) You also may want to use a length of dental floss or string (8-9 inches), to act as a plumb line.

Many photos are provided as examples within the text. To expand your opportunity to practice, I recommend that you study photos of clients and friends, figures in textbooks, pictures in magazines and photos of your own body. When possible, it is good to have four views: front, right side, back, left side. The client should be wearing clothing that enables you to see body contours.

We will use two categories for observation:

1) **Alignment**: The placement and the relationships of body parts, to each other and to the whole body, with respect to a plumb line.

2) **Dimension**: The internal volume, mass or shape of body segments or of the body as a whole. The amount and orientation of the three dimensions of length, depth, and width have great significance on body shape and function.

Following the simple-to-complex format, we will begin assessing these two categories separately, and then see how they affect each other simultaneously.

As I look at all the new content I have added to this edition, I realize it is a progression of my discoveries over 56 years of teaching. My hope is that this progression of content will move your skill sets forward easily and prepare you for Chapters 8 to 10, which cover Aston Theory and Principles.

Pre-test A

In order to appreciate your progress while working through this manual, you may find it helpful to record what, and how, you are seeing now for comparison later. Take a moment to look at the following photo and write down what you see. Use an extra sheet, if necessary.

Answer these questions.

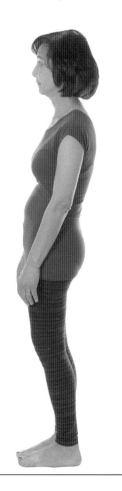

1) What do you see?

2) What do you think this person's complaints might be?

3) What areas might you address in a session or lesson and why?

Notes:

_____

_____

_____

_____

_____

_____

Pre-test B

For your learning and personal application, have a friend photograph you from four different views plus your casual stance.

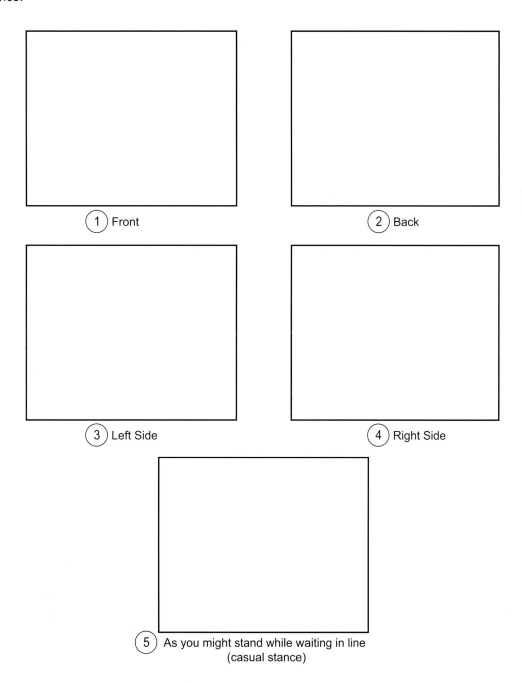

1) Front

2) Back

3) Left Side

4) Right Side

5) As you might stand while waiting in line
(casual stance)

Include your photo series here and, with yourself as the subject, make the same observations and answer the same questions as in Pre-test A (on the previous page).

Introduction

A lot of information can be gained by looking at the body's skeletal landmarks and plumb line. I want to add to that perspective with the concept of seeing all the body's segments as three-dimensional, and how the influences of alignment (placement), dimension (shape) and asymmetry must be included in an assessment.

Alignment includes the placement of the body segments in space, in three-dimensional relationship to one another, as well as to the whole body. We will expand this idea in the next few chapters.

Being able to assess the alignment of the whole body helps us understand primary and secondary contributors to a particular individual's symptoms. Sometimes it is easy to imagine that all people who have the same symptoms share the same body patterns of alignment and might therefore benefit from the same treatment. These two people have low back pain, which is a common complaint. Do they look the same?

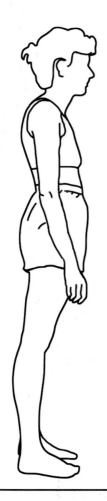

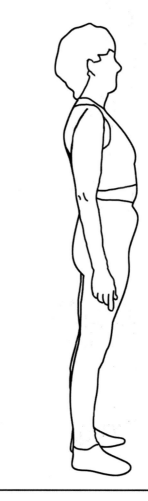

It is important to see that although these people share the same complaint, each pattern adds stress to the back in a different way. A different treatment protocol will be needed to match these two unique patterns.

Alignment and geometric shapes

(**Note**: The majority of the photos in this book show the clients and students demonstrating their 'before' session photos. While their patterns might be exaggerated, it also makes it easier for you to see the patterns.)

Common patterns of alignment

Observe the following common patterns of alignment.

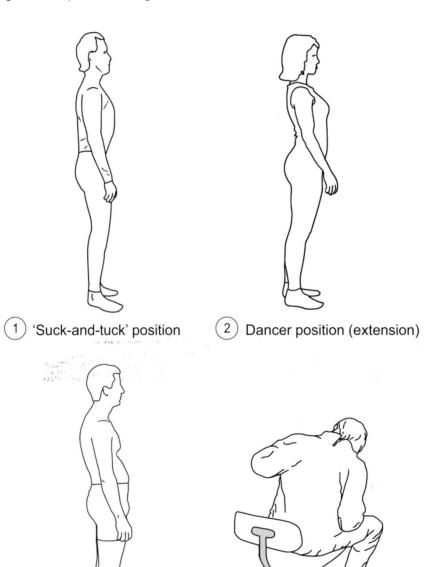

1. 'Suck-and-tuck' position   2. Dancer position (extension)

3. Slouched posture (flexion)   4. A dentist's position (rotation)

Many of these patterns have been learned in order to achieve a specific result. Although they may be effective for the desired goal, they may also result in certain unwanted consequences elsewhere in the body. Some of the adverse consequences are outlined below.

1) Suck-and-tuck position

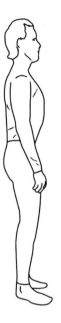

Action
Suck in abdomen.
Tuck pelvis under.

Purpose
To stabilize the spine.
To improve posture.

Consequences
Possible compression and a decrease in the range of movement of the hip and spine.
Moves trunk and pelvis alignment behind midline of hips and legs.

2) Dancer position (extension)

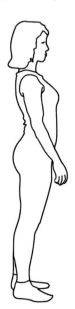

Action
Lift up chest.

Purpose
To elongate the aesthetic line.
To lift off the legs.

Consequences
Stretching the front of the chest.
Possible compression in lower back, which decreases the shock absorption through the spine. This would be a negative consequence for a ballet dancer.

3) Slouched posture (flexion)

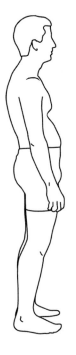

Action
Relax the trunk.

Purpose
To let go, be casual, relieve stress.

Consequences
Compression in the chest, decreased breath, increased pressure in the abdomen and low back.

4) A dentist's position (rotation)

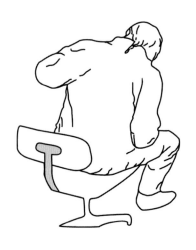

Action
Rotate body segments around center of body.

Purpose
To negotiate the patient, chair and task.

Consequences
Bending without adequate support and prolonged, uneven stress on right and left sides of body and trunk compression affects dexterity of fingers and hands and spinal rotation.

Clearly, each isolated action influences the whole-body pattern. This book will provide a framework for understanding the body as a whole system.

Three planes

The body can be divided into three planes. We will look at each of these planes separately, then combine them to give a simultaneous three-dimensional (3D) description of the alignment, since any real analysis of a 3D object must include all three planes. The body is three-dimensional and therefore, if an optimal change to a body segment occurs, we need to take into account its effect within all three planes. We must consider that a simple change in one plane in one body segment will also affect all other segments of the body, in all three planes.

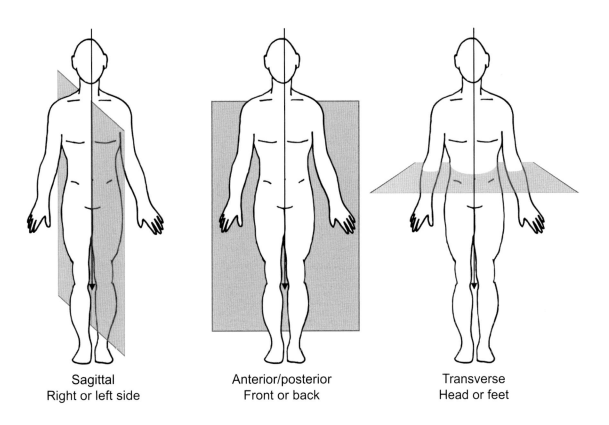

Sagittal	Anterior/posterior	Transverse
Right or left side	Front or back	Head or feet

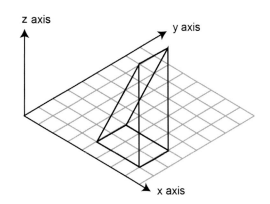

Two-dimensional

y axis

x axis

Three-dimensional

z axis

y axis

x axis

Alignment and geometric shapes

Let's simplify this even more, by looking at six views of the body.

1) The anterior view – from the front.

2) The posterior view – from the back.

3) The right view – from the right side (sagittal).

4) The left view – from the left side (sagittal).

5) The bird's eye view – overhead view of the body (transverse).

6) The worm's eye view – view from the floor, beneath the feet (transverse).

When we observe just one view, we can see two of the three relationships:

1) Front or back views: we can observe right to left (R–L) placement, and high to low placement.

2) Right or left side views: we can observe anterior to posterior (A–P) placement, and high to low placement.

3) Overhead (bird's eye view): we can observe anterior to posterior (A–P) placement, and right to left (R–L) placement.

4) From feet up (worm's eye view): we can observe anterior to posterior (A–P) placement, and right to left (R–L) placement.

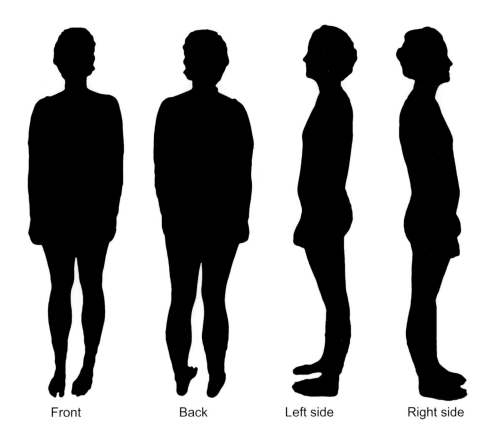

Front   Back   Left side   Right side

1) From the front and back views, what do you imagine to be this client's complaint or focus for a session?

2) Now, look at the two side views. Do you still have the same focus?

Possible theories:

1) You are drawn to the client's left leg and hear that she had to wear a brace on her left leg at night time when she was two years old. This was to correct her extreme external rotation of that leg.

2) Or, from the side view, you are drawn to her strong hyperextension pattern at both knees.

3) Or, from the front view, perhaps the fact that she looks shorter or more compressed on her right side at her knee, hip, chest to shoulder.

4) Or maybe she expressed her history of feeling self-conscious and letting her chest sink down, so she felt more hidden. You might wonder if it is her chest that pushes down on her abdomen and pelvis, which then pushes the lower legs back.

5) Or maybe she described her passion for being a pitcher on a softball team and how she plants her left foot to help control her right pitching arm.

6) Or you are drawn to her front view, with her shoulders rolled in, her legs rolled in, her chest narrow in front and wide in the back.

7) Or you might be influenced by her comment that one teacher tried to correct her posture by having her 'reach for the sky hook'. She hated it and hopes she won't ever have to do that again!

Oh my! Where does one begin?
LET'S GET STARTED!

Alignment and geometric shapes

Abstract shapes

To train our seeing, let's begin with taking a look at these abstract shapes.

Pay attention to their difference in shape and size.

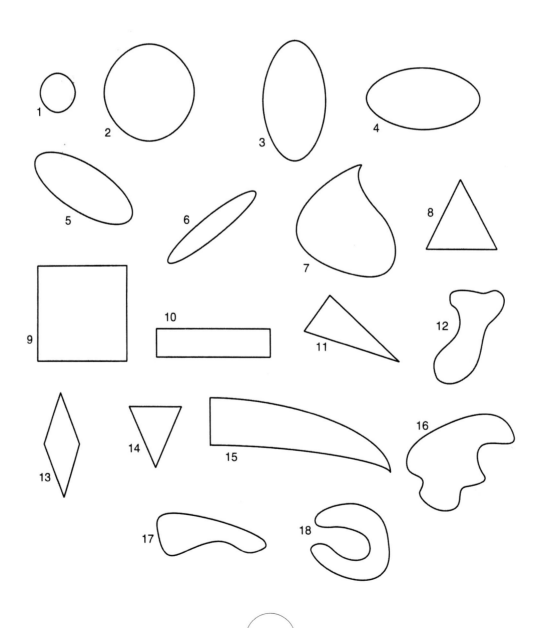

Identifying geometric centers

The spatial geometric center of an object is the **centroid**. When an object is asymmetrical, its center point is toward the larger end. Look at each of these shapes and determine the location of the center of each shape. Place a dot where you think is the spatial center point.

Exercise 2.1

As you glance at the shapes, you will begin to get a sense of how to visually find this center point. Place a transparency over these shapes or use a pencil to locate and mark the geometric center of each shape.

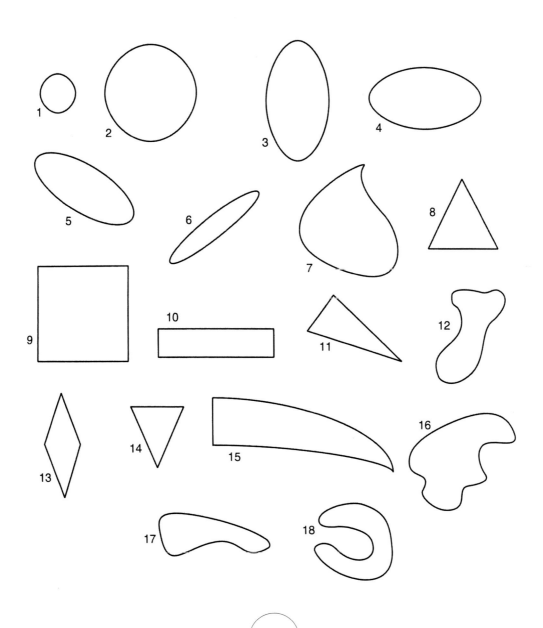

Placement

In examining the alignment of body segments, we first look at the placement of the geometric centers, then at the relationship of the segments or geometric centers to each other. Keeping the three planes in mind, we could say that the placement of one part is right or left, up or down, anterior (front) or posterior (back), to the other.

Exercise 2.2

First, locate and mark the geometric center of each shape in the pairs below.

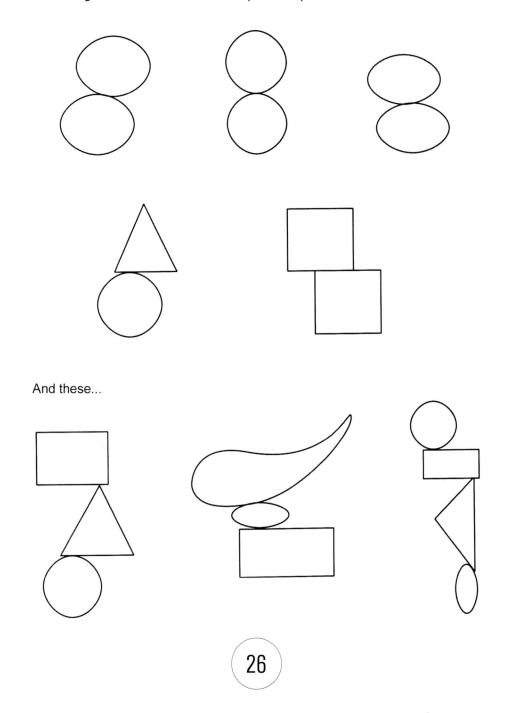

And these...

Now, lay tracing paper over the page and draw lines to connect the center points of these pairs of shapes. Draw the lines and then look at the lines by themselves, on the tracing paper.

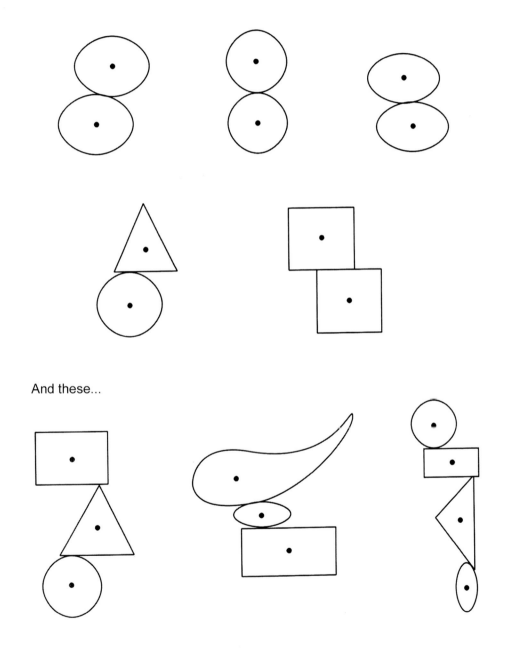

And these...

Alignment and geometric shapes

Exercise 2.3

In these irregularly shaped objects, consider the placement of the geometric centers in relation to each other and to the horizontal line of the 'floor'.

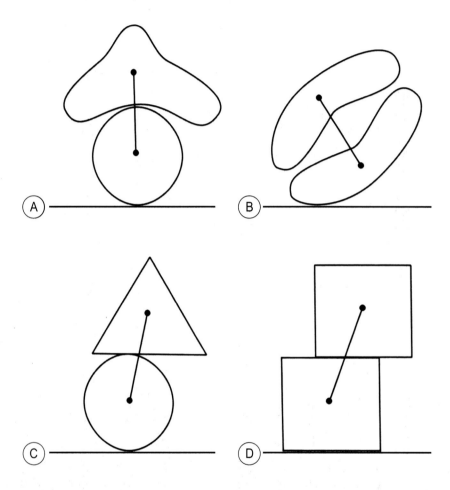

In **A** and **B**: If you begin by looking at the lower shape resting on the floor – then the upper shape is centered left of the lower shape.

In **C** and **D**: The upper shape is centered to the right of the lower shape.

Because of the position of the upper to the lower shape, notice that all four examples are at slightly different angles to each other.

Notation of placement

It is useful to transfer your observations and assessments to the patient's chart without the time-consuming narrative style. These notations can assist your problem-solving during a session and they serve to remind you to compare changes from session to session. They also are useful in writing reports and communicating to your client and other practitioners. In order to make this information easily accessible and visually clear for you and other therapists, we will look at several methods of notating. You will discover what is most useful to you. The following figures show a simple way to quickly notate intersegmental relationships from the right to left perspective.

Symbols

First, place dots to locate the geometric center of each segment. Next, designate a reference point by placing an X that is centered either above the top segment or below the bottom segment. Arrows can then be used to denote the direction of displacement. The distance of placement off-center from the segment below (or above) determines the length of the arrow.

In this example, we start with the reference point (X) at the bottom:

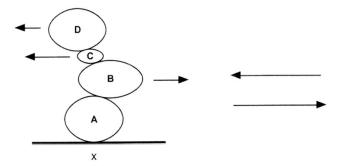

The length of the arrows designates the amount of segmental displacement in relation to the segment immediately above it (when starting from the bottom) or below it (when starting from the top). As you can see, **B** is displaced to the right of **A**, **C** is displaced to the left of **B**, and **D** is also displaced, to the left of **C**.

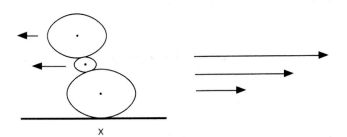

In this example, notice that the middle segment arrow is longer, as its center is further left of the bottom segment.

Alignment and geometric shapes

Exercise 2.4

In relationship to the starting point X, which is segment 1:

1) 2 is placed to the left of 1.

2) 3 appears slightly left, over 2.

3) 4 is more right of 3.

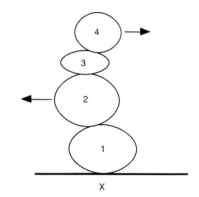

Whether you start from the top or the bottom, X marks the reference point. Since the arrows indicate displacement from the first segment, there is no arrow at the reference point segment. **And there is no arrow when the segment is centered over another.**

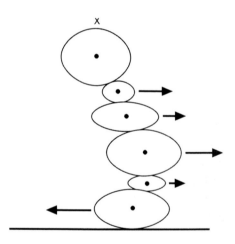

This assessment starts from the top and goes down. There is no arrow on the starting point segment – it is the reference.

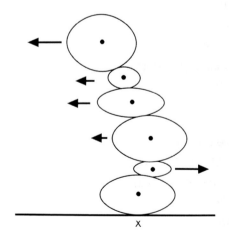

Here is the same pattern, only this assessment starts from the bottom and goes up. There is no arrow on the starting point segment – it is the reference.

Notice the difference in reading this pattern, from top to bottom and bottom to top. We need to be aware of both patterns, as the consequences on a body would be quite different from bottom up, or from top to bottom.

Outlining segments from photographs

Exercise 2.5

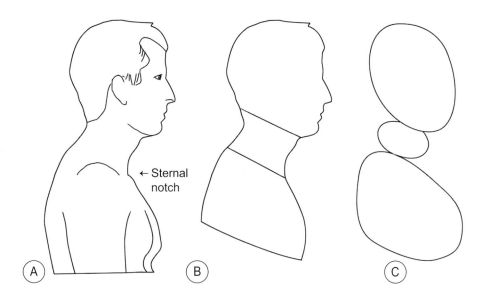

← Sternal notch

Starting with the illustration (A):

- Observe the illustration: upper chest, neck, head. Notice that drawing **B** (outlined body segments) outlines the right side of his chest, from the right view, and does not include the left side of his chest.

On the outline (B):

- Add dots to designate geometric centers (the centroids).
- Connect the dots to observe placement changes. That is, the zig-zag of the line moving left or right of center.

On the ball body (C):

- Add dots for the position of geometric centers, then connect with lines, to observe placement changes.
- Add your reference point X to the **bottom**, then add arrows to notate direction and amount of displacement for each segment.

- Using a different colored pencil or tracing paper, add your reference point X to the **top**, then add arrows to notate direction and amount of displacement for each segment, from this opposite direction.

To recap the notation process:

1) Outline body segments.

2) Add dots, to show geometric centers.

3) Connect the dots with lines.

4) Look at the angle changes, from one segment to the next.

5) Add your X as a reference point.

6) Add arrows to denote which segments move to the left and which move to the right of center, by degree (arrow length).

7) Notice the difference in degree (arrows) when your assessment begins from the reference point (X) at the bottom segment up vs. from the top down.

Alignment and geometric shapes

We've looked at two-dimensional shapes, found their centers and considered their relationships to one another:

1) The shapes.

2) Add geometric centers (dots).

3) Add relationship, connect geometric centers with lines to show segment placement.

4) Add arrows, to show placement of segments to left or right of center.

What happens when we consider other forces acting on these shapes? Forces like weight, effort, gravity, etc.

- Adding weight (larger or heavier shapes will have more force and/or resistance, and will affect the surrounding shapes).

- If segmental boundaries are flexible, surrounding shapes can change the shape of a segment (i.e., heavier shape above will compress and may widen a flexible shape below).

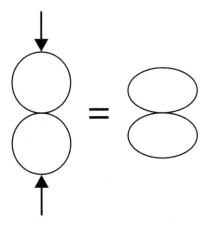

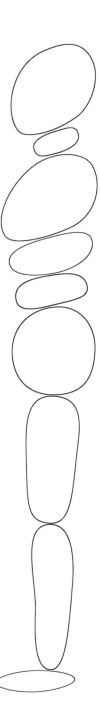

We'll explore these forces and more, as we progress through the book and continue to develop seeing skills.

When I started training physical therapists in my work in 1980, they brought my attention to the term *translation*, to describe shifts. Whichever term fits your understanding better, please use it to refer to the right to left, or anterior to posterior placement of a segment.

I divide the body into nine segments so that we can clearly see how strongly these segments influence one another. I divide the chest into two segments (upper and lower), because of the distinct differences in how people move within the ribcage. While there may be 360 joints in the human body and each one could represent a segment, I propose we look at the body in these nine primary segments.

The nine segments:

1) Head

2) Neck

3) Upper chest

4) Lower chest

5) Abdomen/lumbar area

6) Pelvis

7) Upper leg

8) Lower leg

9) Foot

Three more segments will be added when we include the arms.

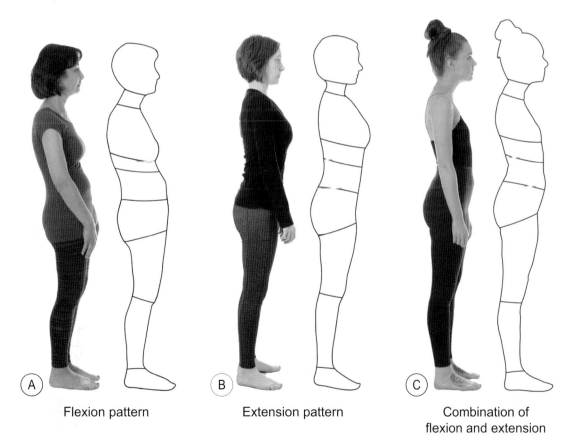

(A) Flexion pattern

(B) Extension pattern

(C) Combination of flexion and extension

The common pattern in example **A** is: (1) upper ribs flexed down, (2) lower ribs may also be flexed. In **B**, the upper and lower ribs are extended up. In **C**, the upper ribs are flexed down, and lower ribs are extended up.

Seeing alignment shifts from the side

Body landmarks in side view

To look at the body segments more three-dimensionally, we begin by focusing on the nine segments (without the arms, initially), using landmarks as divisions.

The following landmarks give us reference points to observe the placement of each segment in relation to adjoining segments, and the angle of segmental relationships *(tilts)* in the side view.

The landmark reference progresses to outlining the segments, then to notating the assessment on a ball body diagram.

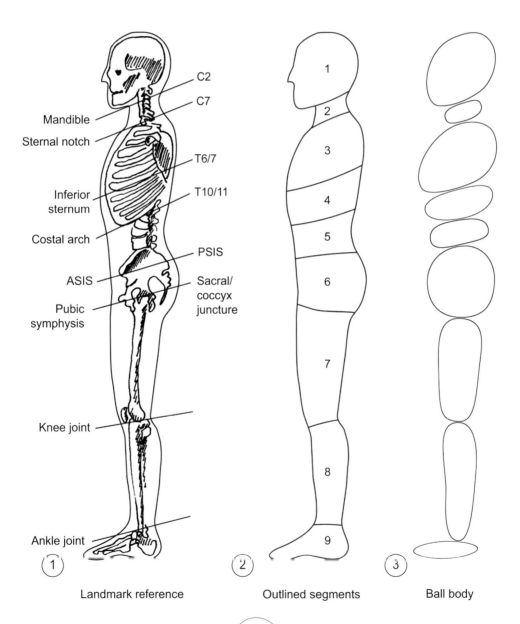

| Landmark reference | Outlined segments | Ball body |

Ball body chart and landmarks – drawing the nine segments

I created the ball body as a quick and easy way to notate the nine body segments. Observe the progression of illustrations below, to see how you begin with landmarks, trace the segments, then notate your findings on the ball body and, eventually, on the body chart.

Progress through these five steps for your learning now. Once you are able to notate the body pattern quickly and accurately, you will not need to go through them all each time.

1) Head

2) Neck

3) Upper chest

4) Lower chest

5) Abdomen/lumbar area

6) Pelvis

7) Upper leg

8) Lower leg

9) Foot

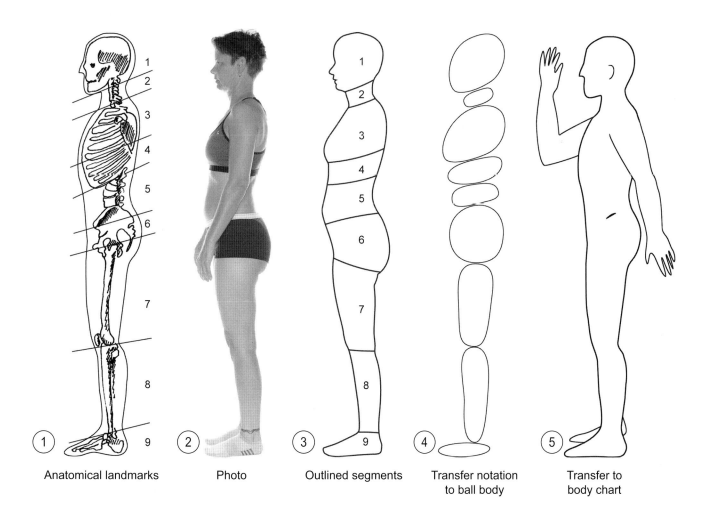

| Anatomical landmarks | Photo | Outlined segments | Transfer notation to ball body | Transfer to body chart |

Seeing alignment shifts from the side

Transferring notations to the ball body

1) Start with the photo: observe the pattern.

2) We've outlined the nine body segments for you, using the landmarks on p. 34.

3) Add your centroids (dots).

4) Connect the dots with lines. Observe the relative anterior–posterior placement of all nine segments.

5) Transfer notations of arrows to the ball body chart.

6) Add the relative length of arrows to demonstrate degree of anterior–posterior displacement.

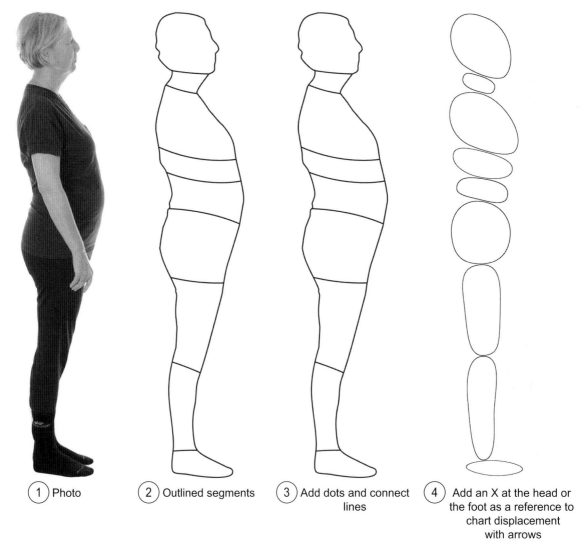

(1) Photo   (2) Outlined segments   (3) Add dots and connect lines   (4) Add an X at the head or the foot as a reference to chart displacement with arrows

Observing your arrow notations, you can see segments placed and displaced in opposite directions. These counter-shifts create shear forces between those segments.

Practice

In your notations, the use of longer and shorter arrows helps demonstrate the relative distance of displacement between one segment and another.

Look at the following photos and compare each to its outline drawing, which also demonstrates the placement of the nine body segments. This exercise of outlining body segments can assist you to quickly identify the body pattern.

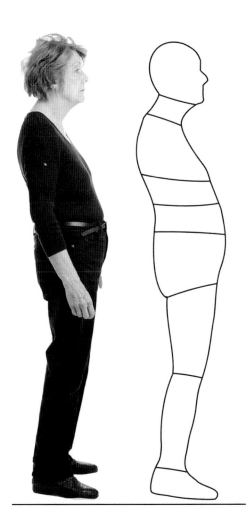
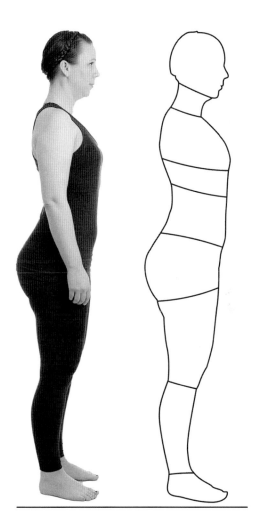

The ball body in nine segments

Continue to train your visual assessment skills by outlining the segments first, then transferring notations to a ball body drawing. Train your eye to see placement relationships, from segment to segment.

Exercise 3.1

1) Look at this body in the photo and its shape, in the outlined form.

2) Using landmarks, add the nine segments to the outline.

3) Add an X at head or foot as a reference point, notate your findings on the ball body.

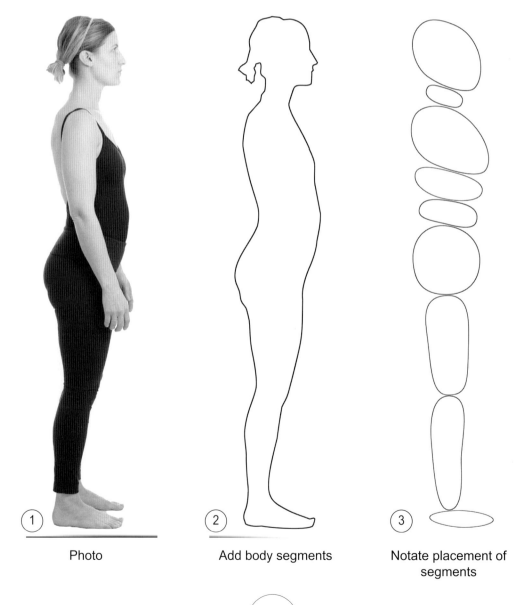

① Photo

② Add body segments

③ Notate placement of segments

Practice

Notate the center alignment in the photos (**1**) onto the drawing (**2**), then mark degree of anterior to posterior (A–P) displacement on the ball body drawing (**3**).

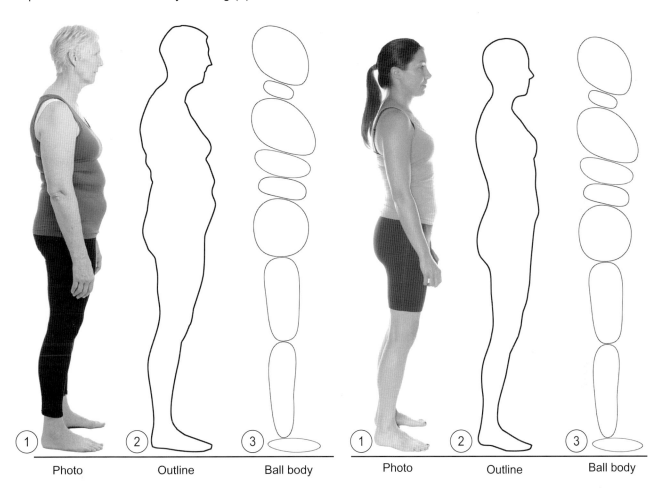

① Photo   ② Outline   ③ Ball body

① Photo   ② Outline   ③ Ball body

After you have made your marks, cover each photo and outlined body drawing and look at your notation by itself. Visualize the alignment of the body you have notated. Uncover the photo and see how well your notes have enabled you to picture this client.

This would be a good time for you to see if you can position your posture to approximate the anterior–posterior relationship of your notations by putting this pattern onto your own body.

Notice which markings were missing or misleading. Alter your notation so that you can reproduce the alignment accurately without the photo. Refining your system of notation will enable you to compare accurately the alignment of a client from one session to the next and to document progress over time.

Exercise 3.2

Complete this exercise for each body shown below.

1) On the first photo, outline the segments.

2) Mark the geometric centers.

3) Connect the centers with lines.

4) Mark arrows for placement of segments in relation to each other, starting from the foot up or head down.

5) Compare your notations to the second photo. How accurate were you?

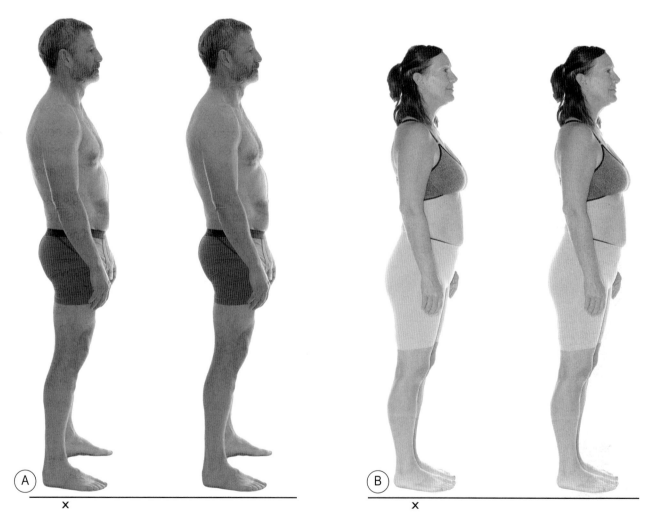

Sometimes, our eye can miss the subtle relationships while being drawn to the obvious ones. This outlining exercise will train your eye to see the placement of all nine body segments and make their relationships to each other more obvious.

Exercise 3.3

Observe the following photos and sketches. Outline the body segments, then notate the positional relationships. Start with the X for the reference point. The foot is the most weight-bearing segment. Then all segments above it are in relation to the placement of the X at the foot.

1) Outline the segments.

2) Mark X to identify the reference point.

3) Notate the placement of each segment with arrows.

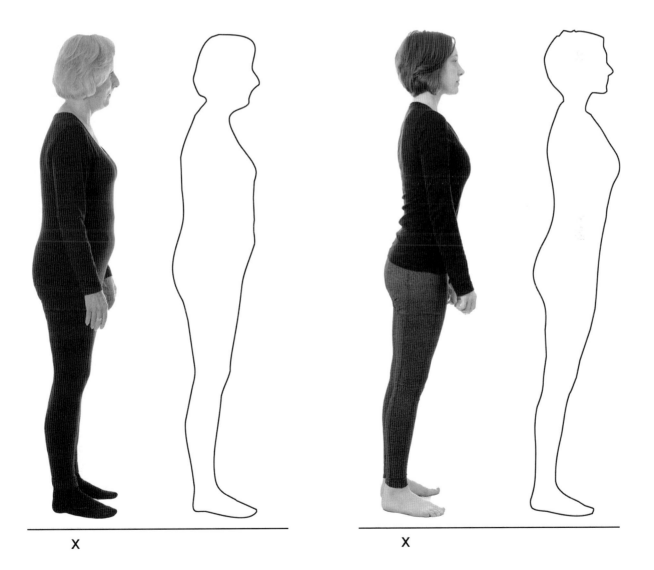

X   X

Exercise 3.4

Reverse your starting point. Perhaps a client comes in having had a severe whiplash at neck and head. Now, notate the same two people, starting from the reference point X placed at the head, down to the feet.

1) Outline the segments.

2) Mark X to identify the reference point.

3) Notate the placement of each segment with arrows.

4) Compare the difference between this top-down notation (X at the head) with the bottom-up version (X at the foot) from the previous exercise.

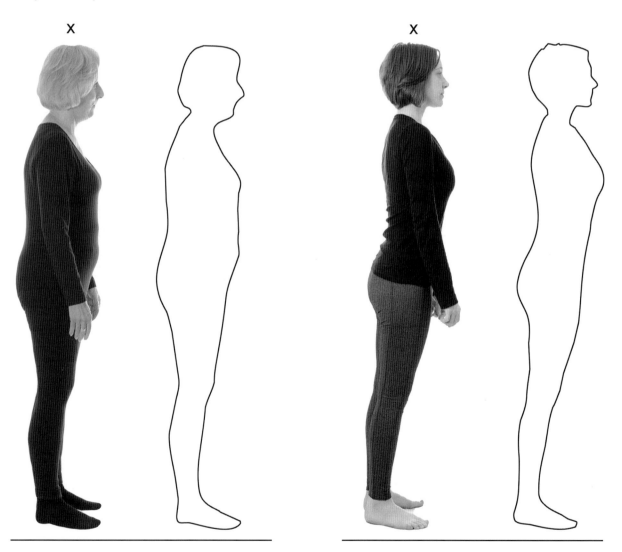

Transferring notations from photos to body charts

Some therapists use photographs to track changes in a client's posture. These can serve as a useful measure of progress and a visual reference for study. The notations we have just worked with can be useful if they are marked directly on the photographs in a patient's file.

Whether you are using photos or notating the person while he or she is standing in front of you, it is useful to transfer your observations to a body chart. This can be done by putting the same notations of placement onto a body chart, like the one shown below.

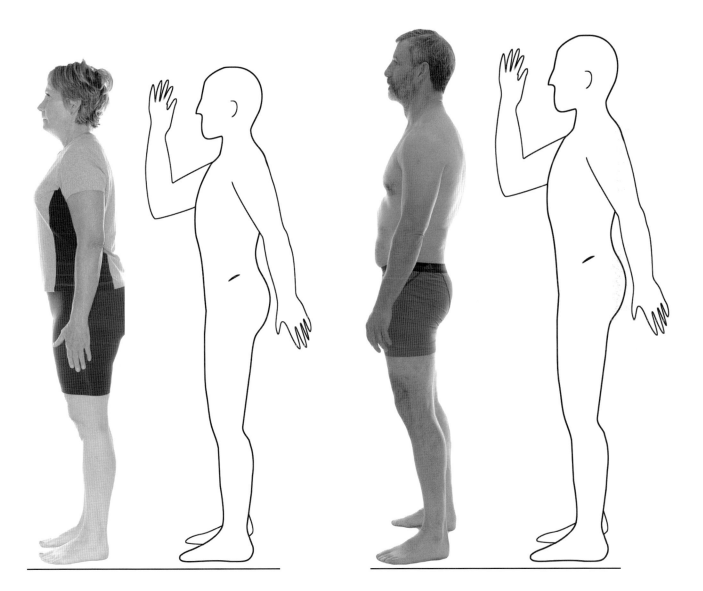

Plumb line – side view

The definition of the plumb line is a 90-degree line perpendicular to the Earth. The traditional use of the plumb line (in the side view) intersects the ear, shoulder, lumbar spine, hip, knee and ankle.

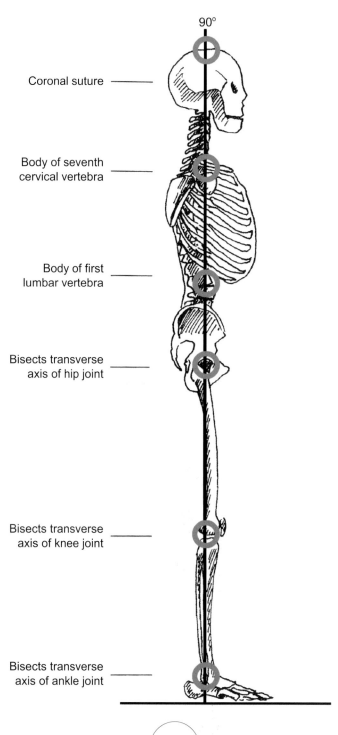

90°

Coronal suture

Body of seventh cervical vertebra

Body of first lumbar vertebra

Bisects transverse axis of hip joint

Bisects transverse axis of knee joint

Bisects transverse axis of ankle joint

By adding a plumb line to a client's photo from the floor, through the ankle and up, we have an additional tool that can quickly determine a body's spatial relationship.

Demonstration

Below is a demonstration of notating in the following sequence:

1) Segments are outlined.

2) An X is marked to notate placement of the reference point.

3) The plumb line is drawn. (Tip: use a length of dental floss or string to establish the location, then use a ruler or straight edge to draw a line perpendicular to the floor and up through the ankle.)

4) The horizontal arrows are drawn to designate placement of segments anterior or posterior to the plumb line.

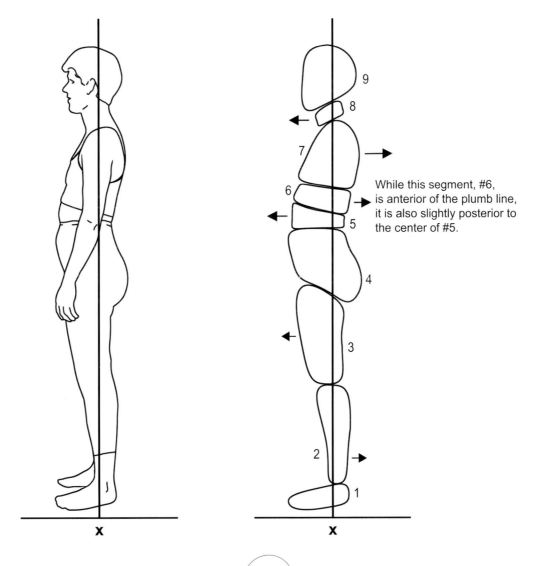

While this segment, #6, is anterior of the plumb line, it is also slightly posterior to the center of #5.

Practice combining notations of alignment

Let's review the concepts and skills we have learned up to this point. Using the following three photos:

1) Outline the nine segments.

2) Mark the geometric centers.

3) Mark an X to designate the starting point at the feet or head.

4) Connect the geometric centers.

5) Notate the direction and amount of anterior–posterior displacement with arrows.

6) Compare to the plumb line.

7) Based on the information gained from steps 1 to 6, where is the major point of weight bearing under the foot (toward heel, forefoot)? Place an arrow ↑ to designate the greatest weight-bearing area on the foot.

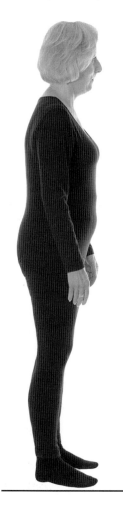 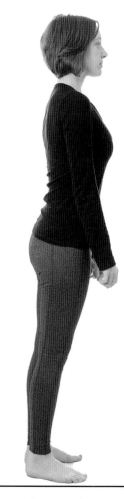 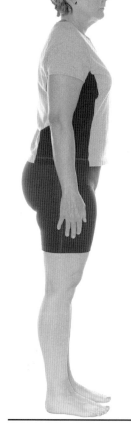

for example

Body charts

Now, go from observing the photo to notating directly onto the body chart. In addition to client notations, many therapists have clients mark areas of pain and injury on body charts. This practice of notating will reveal more information, when you compare your notation to your clients' complaints.

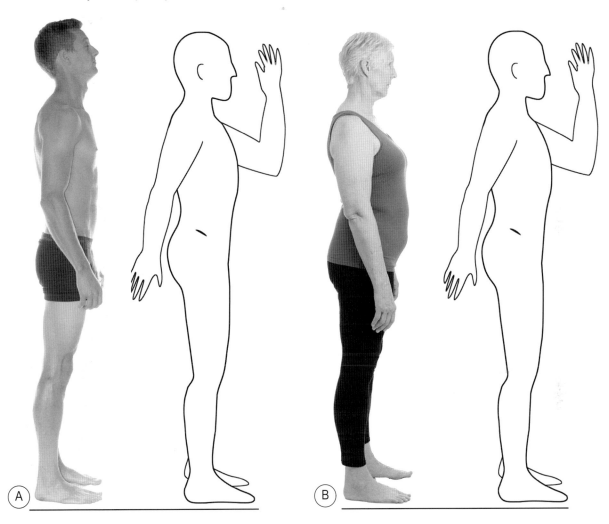

A B

Draw arrows to identify anterior–posterior placement of body segments, and where you see the greatest weight-bearing on the foot.

The body pattern in **A** reveals a common but often missed relationship. The client's neck is forward, but his head is centered back on his neck.

In **B**, the client's neck is aligned more over the posterior placement of the upper chest. The upper chest is back, the neck is a little forward and her head is more central on the neck.

Exercise 3.5

Use these body charts to notate the alignment and weight-bearing shown in photos **A** and **B**. Draw arrows to identify anterior–posterior placement of body segments, and where you see the greatest weight-bearing on the foot.

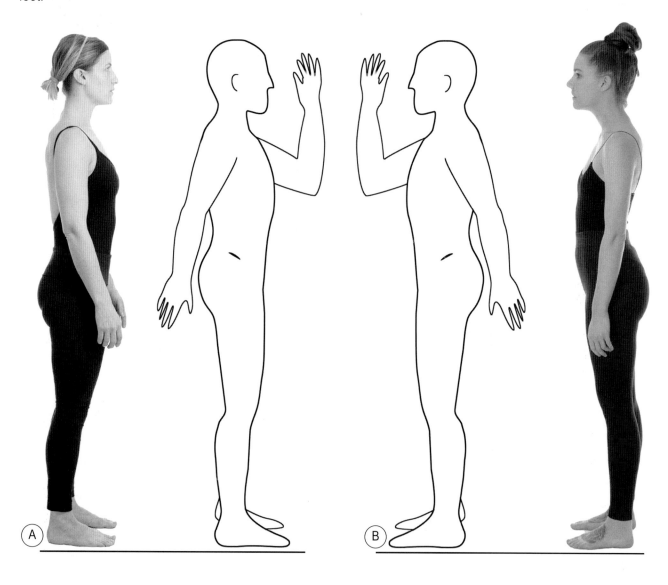

Observe the progression of illustrations to see how the body segments define the ball body.

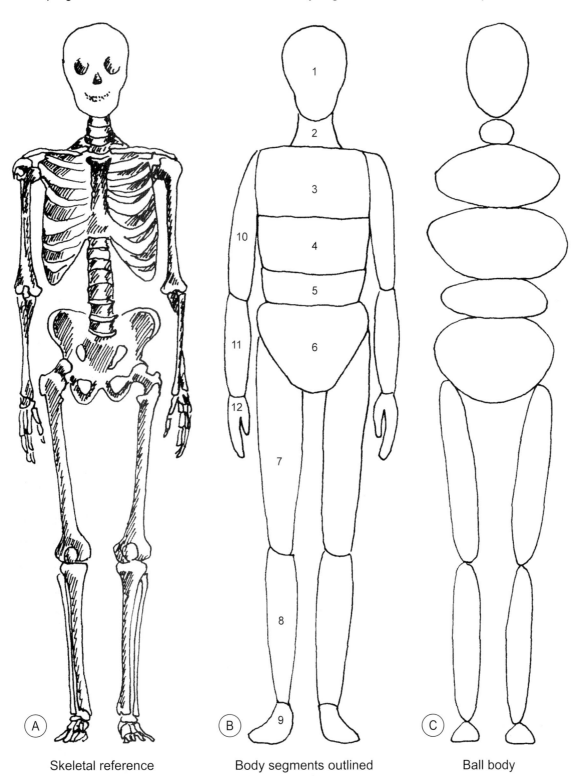

Skeletal reference   Body segments outlined   Ball body

Seeing alignment shifts from the front view

Exercise 4.1

To break down your assessment more specifically, take a piece of paper and cover all the body segments above this woman's feet. Focus on the front view. As you observe the feet, anticipate where you imagine the lower legs to be positioned. Moving your paper one segment at a time, continue up the body to observe each segment and anticipate the position of the next segment above.

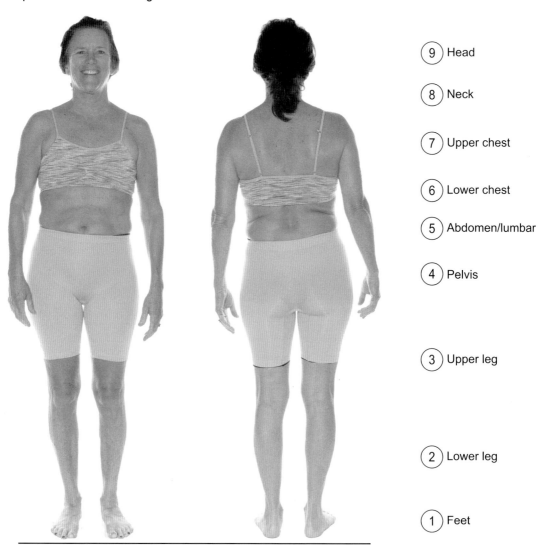

9) Head

8) Neck

7) Upper chest

6) Lower chest

5) Abdomen/lumbar

4) Pelvis

3) Upper leg

2) Lower leg

1) Feet

Viewing the front, were you surprised by the amount her pelvis shifts to the right, and her chest shifts to the left? Can you see how her pattern is even more obvious from the back? Sometimes another view can give you more information.

Covering all body segments and starting from either the bottom or top segments first often reveals more to the eye, or makes displacement more obvious than looking at a whole body at once.

Segmental centers and relationship to placement

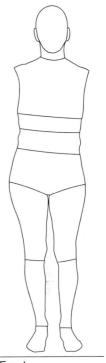

Front

This is the segmented outline of the woman pictured on the previous page.

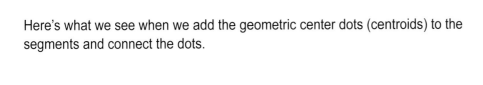

Here's what we see when we add the geometric center dots (centroids) to the segments and connect the dots.

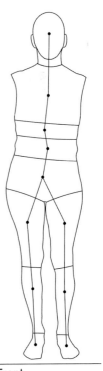

Front

Exercise 4.2

Use your tracing paper to outline the nine body segments on the photo. Add geometric centers to each segment (dots), then connect with lines, to see side to side shifts of segments.

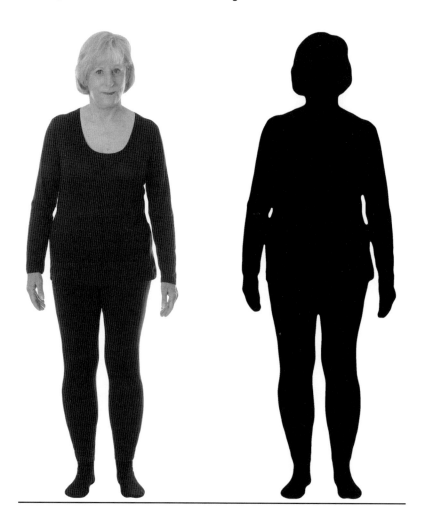

Notation of right to left placement in the frontal plane

Now, let's observe the right to left relationships of the segments to each other in the frontal plane. (This is the same woman from the previous page.)

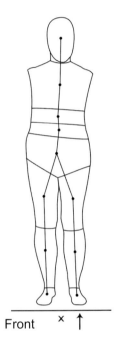

Front   × ↑

The zig-zag line, created by connecting centers, makes the placement obvious.

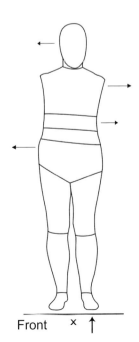

Front   × ↑

We can now progress to documenting placement right or left with arrows. An X marks our reference point, and the ↑ indicates the area of greatest weight-bearing.

Seeing alignment shifts from the front view

Exercise 4.3

A) Observe the three photos below.

1) Outline segments.

2) Mark the geometric centers of each segment.

3) Connect the centers.

4) Starting from the feet and going toward the head, use arrows to notate the right to left placement of each segment in relation to the segment below.

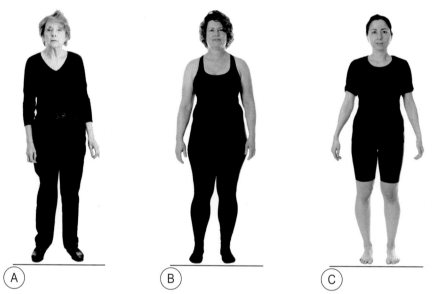

B) Now, transfer your notations to a body chart.

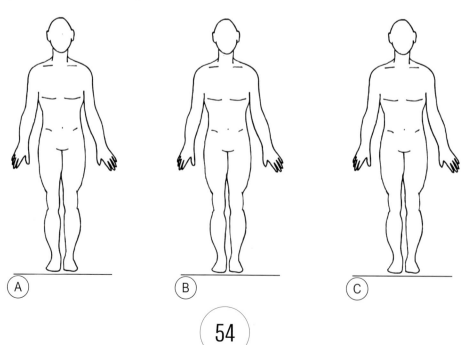

C) Being more specific: starting with the feet, check the length of the arrows you drew on the previous page to notate the placement of each segment, in relation to the segment below. The length of each arrow determines the amount of displacement to the segment below.

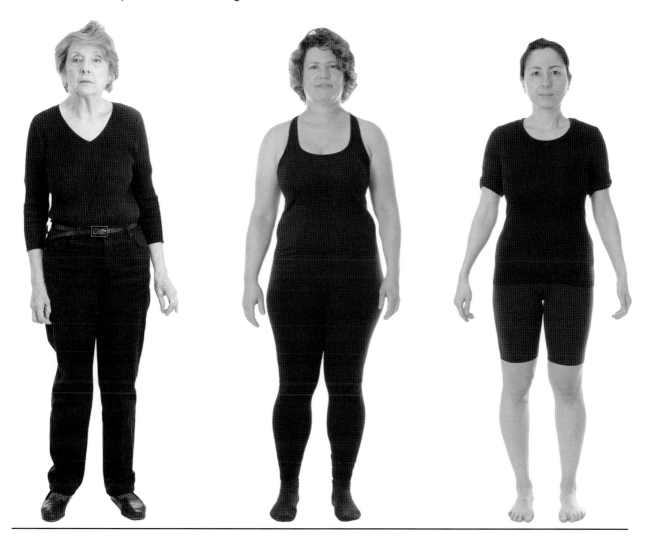

Do the women have their weight mostly on their right foot or their left foot? Use your dental floss (at 90 degrees from the midpoint between the feet) to determine if there is more body mass to the right or left. Use an up arrow (↑) to identify the areas of greatest weight-bearing.

Front plumb line dividing the right and left sides of the body

In reality, most bodies do not demonstrate a pattern where the right and left sides are exactly the same.

Exercise 4.4

Establish the plumb line: hold your dental floss taut and place it midway between the feet, stretched up to the head, perpendicular to the horizontal line.

Place dots where you imagine segmental centers to be for:
a)   Pubic symphysis
b)   Navel
c)   Inferior sternum
d)   Sternal notch

Connect segmental centers (dots) with lines:
a)   Pubic symphysis
b)   Navel
c)   Inferior sternum
d)   Sternal notch

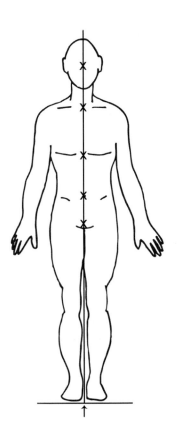

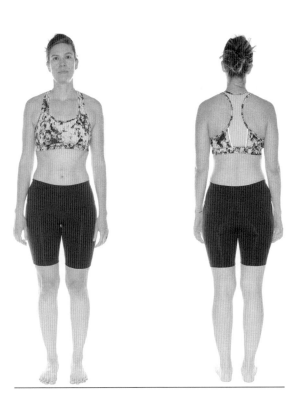

Do you see the same pattern carry through to the back view?

The Central Line

Exercise 4.5

1) Use your dental floss (midway between the feet and 90 degrees to the horizontal line) to identify the plumb line in these photos.

2) Line up the landmarks (pubic symphysis, navel, inferior sternum, sternal notch).

3) Compare these photos with those on the previous page. Which body pattern is more directly aligned?

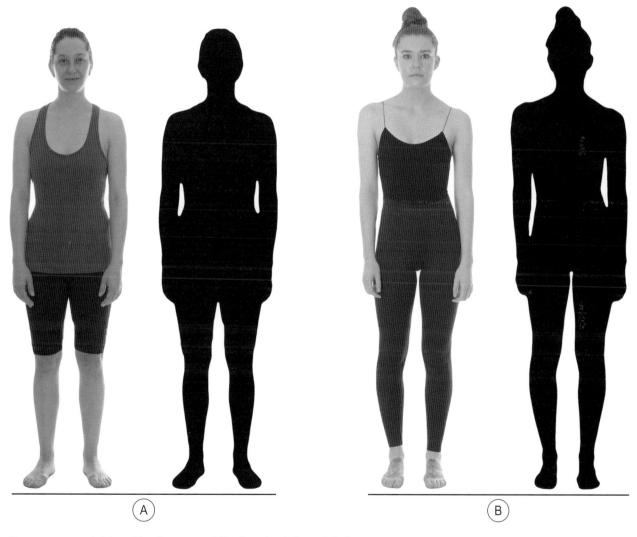

A

B

Is there more weight and body mass shifted to the left or right?

Although both women have their chests shifted right, we can see that most of the body mass of client **A** is shifted to the left and more of the body mass of client **B** is shifted slightly right.

Seeing alignment shifts from the front view

Exercise 4.6

By adding the central line to the drawing of our client below, it is easy to see that the pelvis is placed to her right and the mid and upper trunk are placed to her left.

Use tracing paper to place dots on the following landmarks:
a) Pubic symphysis
b) Navel
c) Inferior sternum
d) Sternal notch
e) Bridge of the nose

Starting with the midpoint between the feet, connect these landmark dots with lines:
a) Pubic symphysis (you will see lower segmental mass placement)
b) Navel
c) Inferior sternum
d) Sternal notch
e) Bridge of the nose

Compare your notation with the drawing.

Where do you think she is bearing most of her weight? On her left foot or her right foot?

I know her pattern, and in this case: the answer is left because the shift of her upper body adds more weight to her left foot. Weight-bearing will become even more obvious when we add rotations, in Chapter 6.

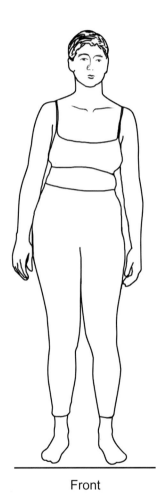

Front

58

I have been suggesting that you take a piece of dental floss and stretch it to create a straight line at 90 degrees to the floor, starting midway between the feet. You can also create a plumb bob, for your evaluation.

Exercise 4.7

This demonstrates how the body adjusts for displacement.

1) Make a plumb bob using dental floss, with a paperclip added to one end, to act as a weight.

2) Set this book upright (standing vertically).

3) Hang the plumb bob in front of each photo, to see the center and the placement of the segments to the right and left.

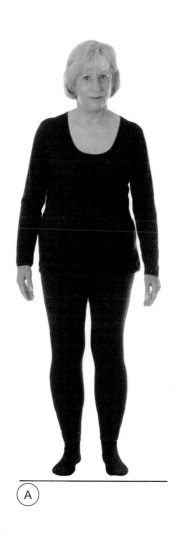

(A)

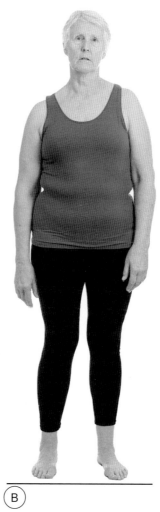

(B)

With your dental floss plumb bob, you can see that woman **A**'s pelvis shifts right and her chest and chin shift left, while woman **B** has more segments shifted to her left.

Notations of weight-bearing on the foot

Placement of all the body segments will determine whether one is centered more over the left or the right foot. This can be notated by placing an arrow under the area that seems to be the center point of most weight-bearing.

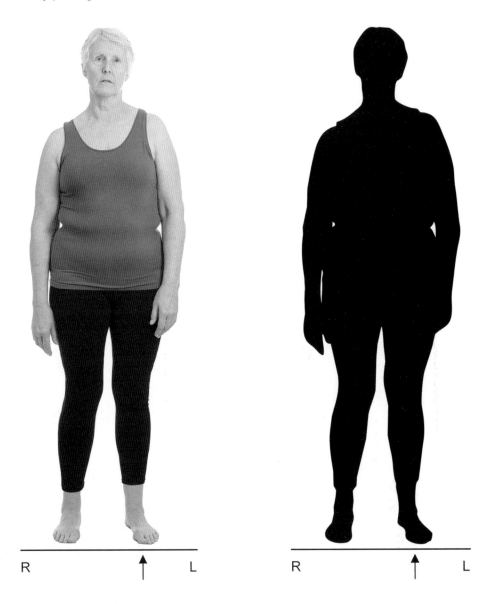

People are often unaware that their body's weight-bearing can be quite uneven from one foot to the other. Additionally, people also have very different areas of weight-bearing on each individual foot, e.g. more weight on the front of one foot, and to the back, inside or outside of the other foot.

I often suggest people use the silhouette feature to see the shape and positioning of the body's mass. We will use silhouettes throughout this book.

Exercise 4.8

To help you determine the greater weight-bearing side.

1) Instruct your client to stand on both feet. Pause. Observe.

2) Then ask them to shift weight to the right side, and maintain this position until he or she feels centered and balanced. Pause.

3) Shift weight back to the middle (center). Pause.

4) Ask them to shift weight to the left side. Pause.

5) Come back to center. Pause.

6) Have the client shift their body weight to the right foot until they can pick up the left foot and then come back to the centered position.

7) From the center position, have the client shift their weight over to the left foot until they can pick up the right foot and then come back to the center.

8) The side that has the least amount of range is usually the side where the person centers most of their weight-bearing.

Just by looking, which side is this client most centered over? Use your dental floss.

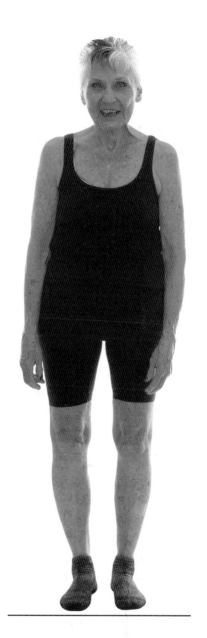

Seeing alignment shifts from the front view

Exercise 4.9

Starting point: generally, start with the feet, because it is the greatest area of weight-bearing.

1) Observe body **A**.

2) Use your dental floss to determine if more body mass appears shifted to the right or left.

3) Notate:

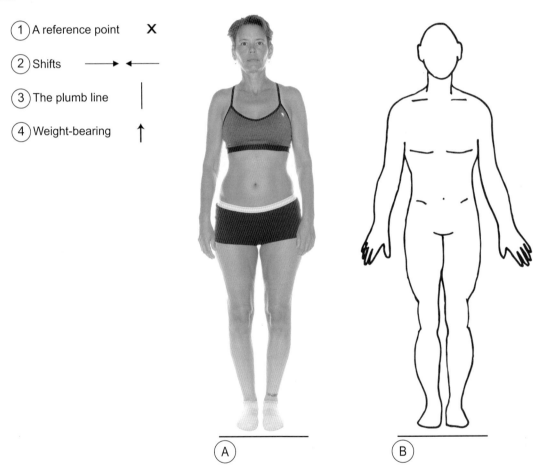

- ① A reference point   **X**
- ② Shifts   ⟶   ⟵
- ③ The plumb line |
- ④ Weight-bearing   ↑

Ⓐ   Ⓑ

4) Place a transparency over the photo (**A**), to notate the segmental shapes within the body.

5) Remove the transparency to see these relationships on the photo, without using your notation marks.

6) Add your notation to the body chart (**B**). As you look at just the notations, do you see the same pattern that caught your eye in photo **A**?

Being able to identify the changes from before to after a session will help you and your client, and will prepare you for the next session.

This is an important skill set to have when educating your client about their own pattern and changes.

CHAPTER 5

Seeing alignment and horizontal tilts from four views

So far we have looked at right and left displacements (shifts) in the frontal plane, and front to back displacements in the transverse plane. Now, in the transverse plane, we'll examine **tilts**. These are the high to low, superior to inferior angles that can generally be observed at joints. Let's identify the position of the different landmark areas for tilts.

Landmarks – front view

Landmark options (descending from the head)

1) Top of head

2) Maxilla*

3) Mandible (inferior border)

4) Top of clavicle**

5) Shoulder joint

6) 6th rib to inferior sternum

7) Costal arch

8) Elbow joint

9) Iliac crest

10) Wrist joint

11) Hip joint

12) Tips of fingers

13) Knee joint

14) Ankle joint

* Mostly you see the angle at the maxilla and the temporomandibular joint (TMJ) to be close to the same; however, with detailed observation, you may identify the maxilla as level, but unevenness at the inferior border of the mandible reveals a strong asymmetry within the joint.

** Sometimes you can observe the clavicle low on one side, yet the humerus high on that same side.

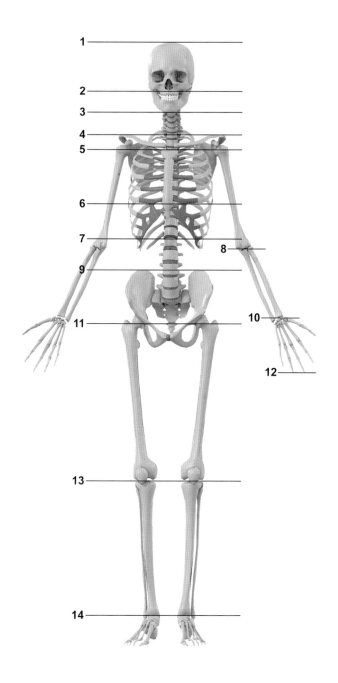

Seeing alignment and horizontal tilts

Connecting landmarks to observe tilt relationships – front view

Exercise 5.1

This exercise helps reveal high to low tilts between right to left sides.

Using a transparency or tracing paper:

1) On the center skeleton below (#2) select from the 14 landmark options (on the previous page) and draw horizontal lines across the body, to connect the landmarks on right and left sides.

2) Observe the line drawing on the far right, which is the same person as the center skeleton. Notice how the right hand being lower matches the tilt at the shoulder.

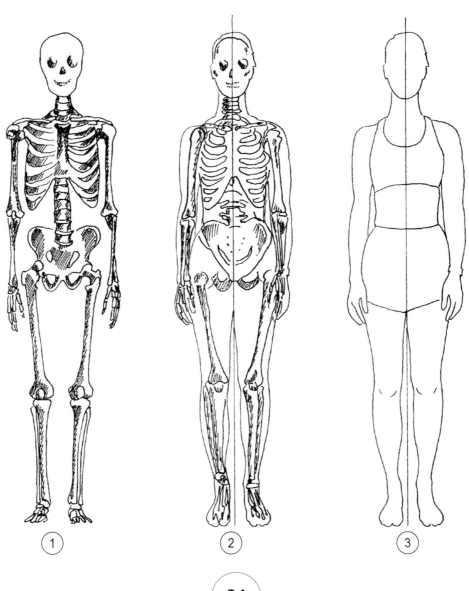

① ② ③

Let's observe a body pattern that is not as symmetrical as that in the last illustration. We have notated the landmarks below demonstrating more obvious displacement.

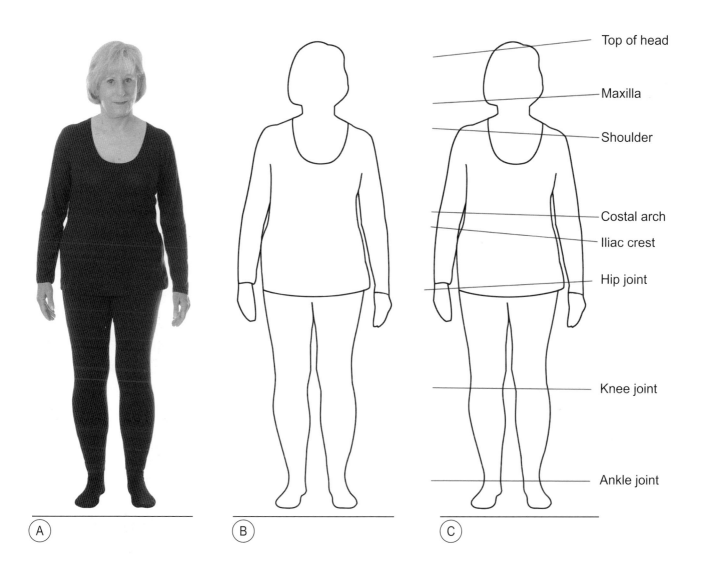

Top of head

Maxilla

Shoulder

Costal arch

Iliac crest

Hip joint

Knee joint

Ankle joint

A   B   C

The right to left unevenness in this drawing (**C**) starts to show us areas of compression (low placement), with other landmarks being stretched (pushed or pulled high).

When the tilt of two lines can intersect, there is usually greater compression between those two segments, on that side. In this case, between her maxilla and right shoulder. This finding may coincide with the client's feedback on the areas of most stress or discomfort.

When we add rotation (in the next chapter), we will see that her right iliac crest is higher because of the rotation.

Seeing alignment and horizontal tilts

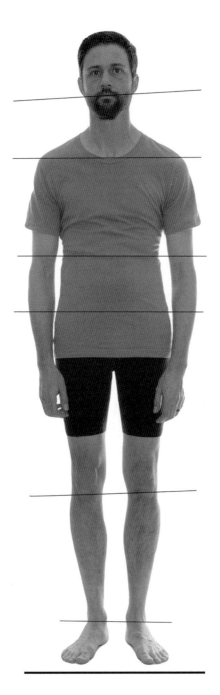 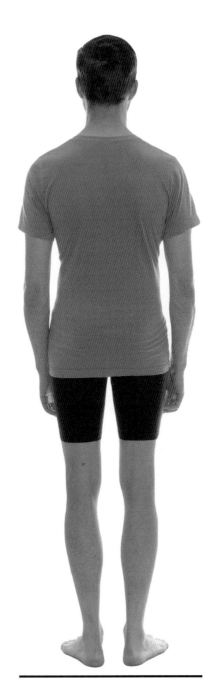

Here is an example of a pattern where the tilts are closer to level, throughout the body. When you observe this client and draw the horizontal landmark lines, you see he looks fairly even right to left.

Exercise 5.2

For both views, draw the horizontal lines connecting the right to left landmarks at the joints. Observe the high to low relationships. Are they the same in both front and back views, or quite different?

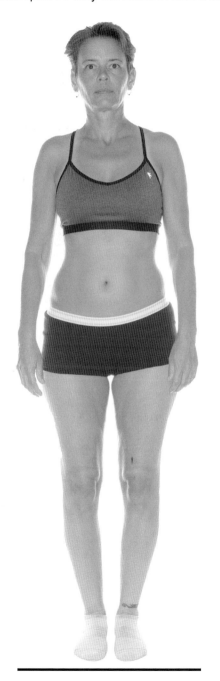 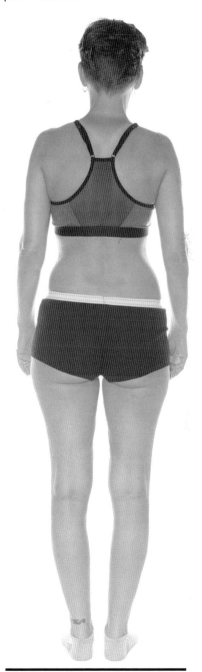

Exercise 5.3

Draw the horizontal lines connecting the right to left landmarks at joints. Observe the high to low relationships. Get some distance from the page and just observe the angles and tilts.

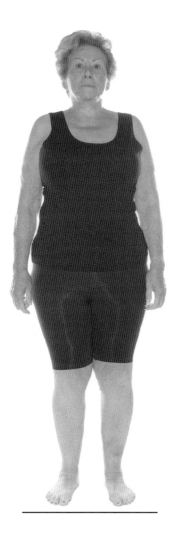 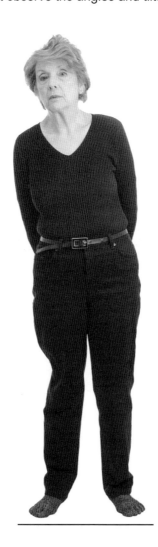 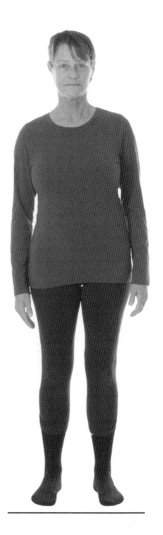

Observing the angles of the tilts reveals the body challenges of compression (low) or stretching (high) at different segments. Often it appears as though the changes in the tilts (from low in one segment to high in the next) show how the body compensates and counter-compensates, to balance the body segments closer to its center, the midline.

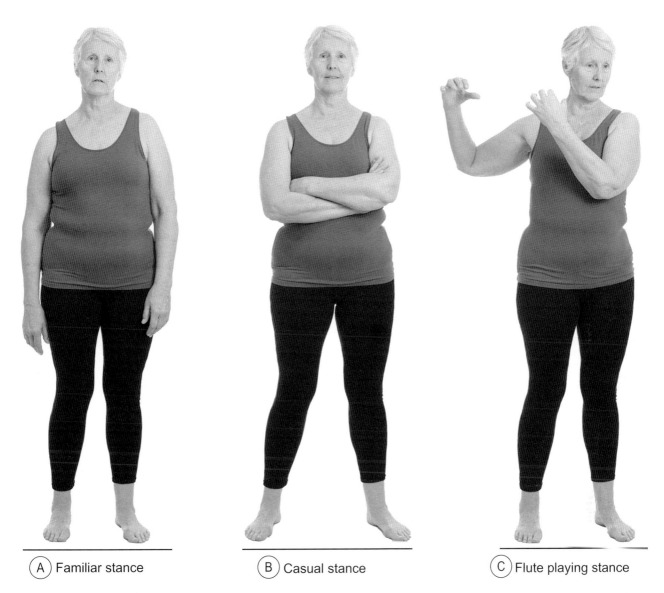

(A) Familiar stance

(B) Casual stance

(C) Flute playing stance

I asked this woman (pictured above) if she had ever done any sport or activity that made her left shoulder high. She said, 'I played flute for many years' (**C**).

This gives added explanation for her familiar stance (**A**) showing the high/low tilt of her head and shoulders, shift of her chest left and more weight on her left foot.

In photo **B**, do your see how crossing her arms decreases her head tilt?

Landmarks – back view

Landmark options (descending from the head)

1) Top of head
2) Occipital ridge
3) C2
4) Top of scapula (C7)
5) Shoulder joint
6) Across T6/7
7) Lowest point of border of the 10th rib
8) Elbow joint
9) Iliac crest
10) Wrist joint
11) Hip joint
12) Tips of fingers
13) Knee joint
14) Ankle joint

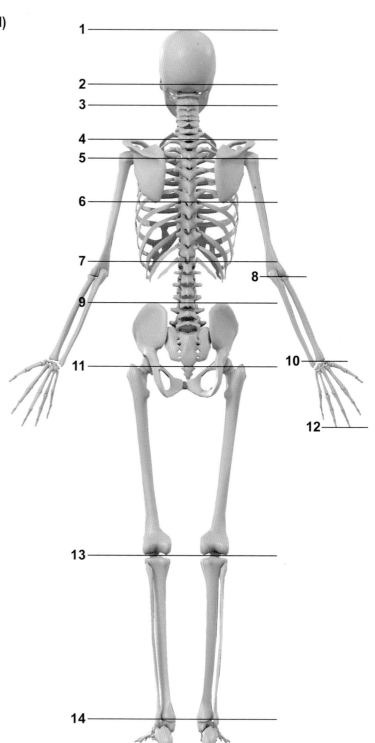

Examples

This client is a trained athlete and very dedicated to her sports and yoga teaching.

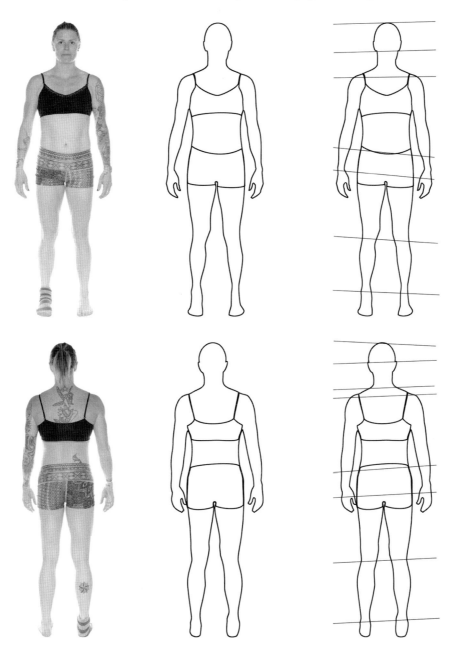

Observe the front and back views:

1) Are the high to low (up to down) patterns as obvious from both views?

2) Are they tilted in the same direction front to back or do they differ?

Connecting landmarks to body segments and ball body – back view

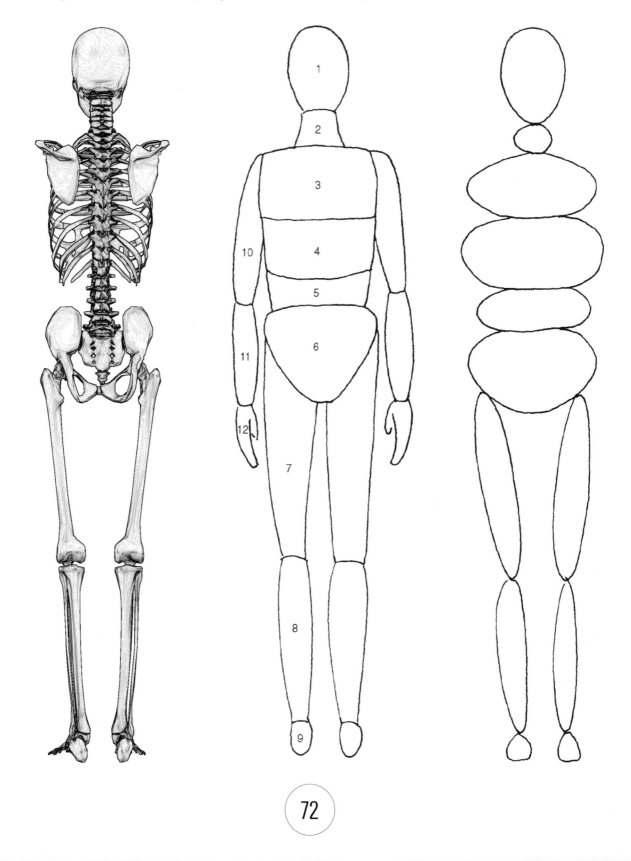

Exercise 5.4

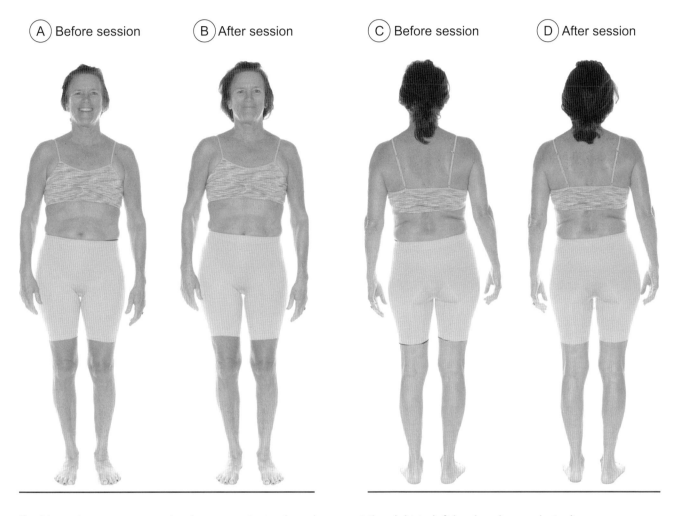

(A) Before session   (B) After session   (C) Before session   (D) After session

1) Use a transparency or tracing paper to mark and connect the right to left landmarks on photo A.

2) Did you skip any landmarks as you were moving up? (Refer to the front and back landmark reference charts, earlier in this chapter.)

3) Overlay your transparency or tracing paper onto B (after session photo), to see if the tilts are the same as A (before session photo).

4) Repeat the exercise with before and after photos, C and D.

Also, does the client have more body mass centered over her left foot or her right foot? Does her weight-bearing seem the same in her after photos?

Combining tilts, shifts and weight-bearing notations

Exercise 5.5

For each example (**A, B** and **C**), select whether the *tilts* or *shifts* draw your attention the most. First, add the notations for your selection (tilts or shifts), then add the notations for the second track. Lastly, add an arrow at the foot, where you see the most weight-bearing.

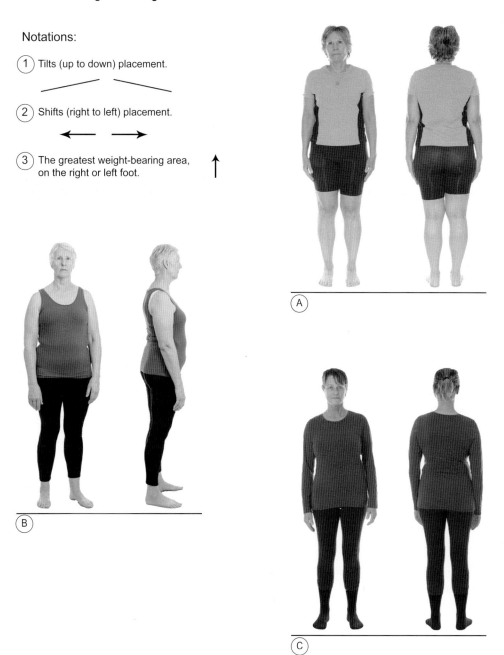

Notations:

1 Tilts (up to down) placement.

2 Shifts (right to left) placement.

3 The greatest weight-bearing area, on the right or left foot.

A

B

C

Notating tilts from the side view

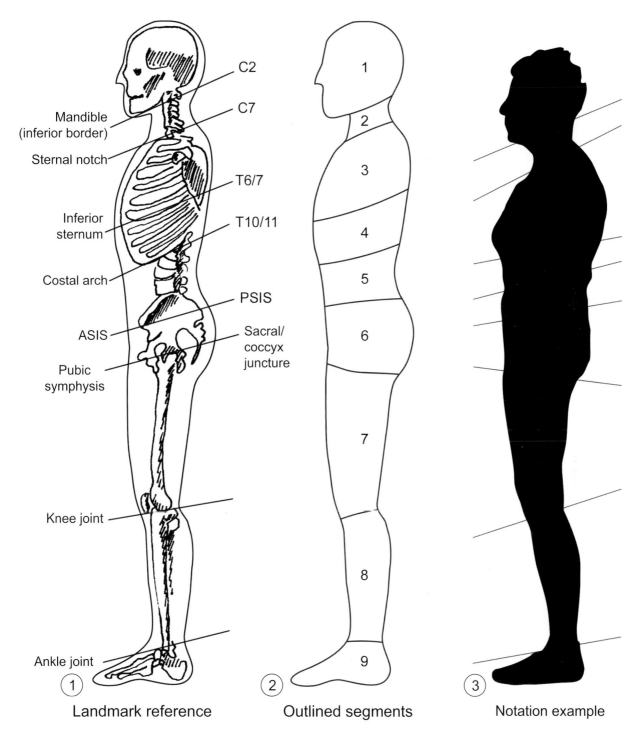

① Landmark reference

Landmark labels:
- C2
- C7
- Mandible (inferior border)
- Sternal notch
- T6/7
- T10/11
- Inferior sternum
- Costal arch
- PSIS
- ASIS
- Sacral/ coccyx juncture
- Pubic symphysis
- Knee joint
- Ankle joint

② Outlined segments

Segments numbered 1–9

③ Notation example

Exercise 5.6

For each example (**A** and **B**), add the tilt and shift notations for the segments that draw your attention the most. Also, add the arrow for perceived weight-bearing on the foot.

Notations:

(1) Tilts (up to down) placement.

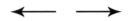

(2) Shifts (anterior to posterior) placement.

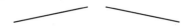

(3) The greatest weight-bearing area, on the front or back foot. ↑

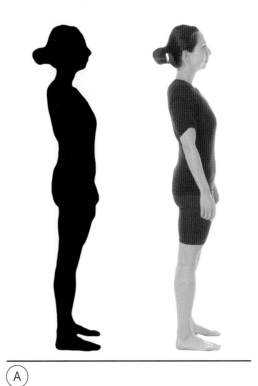

(A)

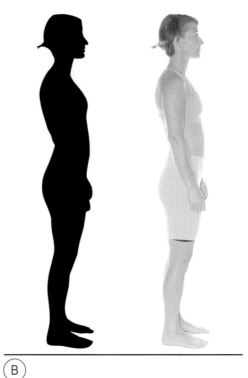

(B)

Combining shifts and tilts of the pelvis – side view

We observed the high to low (tilt) relationships of segments from the front and back views. Let us now examine the tilt of the pelvis (the pelvic tilt) from the side view.

Earlier, we observed the pelvis from the side view, with its anterior to posterior shifts; also from the front and back views, we observed the right to left placement and the high to low placement.

The **difference between shifts and tilts** is an important, and often overlooked distinction. **Shifts** refer to anterior–posterior or right–left placement, in the horizontal plane. **Tilts** refer to angles, seen from front, back or sides, in the superior to inferior or high to low relationships of segments.

In order to determine the tilt of the pelvis, we need to consider the position of the posterior superior iliac spine (PSIS) in relation to the anterior superior iliac spine (ASIS), as the top landmarks. The other landmark we need to identify is the position of the ischial tuberosity to the femur.

- **Neutral:** The pelvis will appear to be positioned more on top of the leg. The angle of the ASIS to PSIS, and the pubic tubercle to the sacral/coccyx juncture, are tilted slightly anterior. This position allows for more freedom of leg motion at the hip joint.
- **Posterior tilt:** This position angles the pelvis back and down, often bringing the ischial tuberosities down on the posterior aspect of the femur. There are many reasons this can occur. Two examples might be from tight posterior pelvic and leg muscles, or the opposite, from low muscle tone.
- **Anterior tilt**: This position usually angles the top of the pelvis, the ASIS/PSIS, anterior and the ischial tuberosities are often lifted up, off the femur. This can occur from short anterior muscles including the psoas and leg muscles.

Examples

In the examples below, the neutral pelvis is angled about 5 degrees forward. The posterior pelvis is about 10 degrees back, and the anterior pelvis is about 25 degrees forward.

For each example, draw a line from the ASIS to the PSIS, and between the pubic symphysis and the sacral/coccyx juncture. Also notate whether the pelvis is shifted forward or back on the leg.

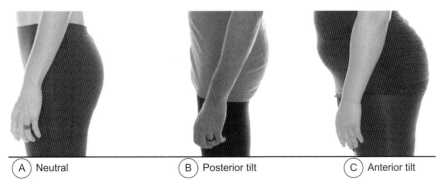

| (A) Neutral | (B) Posterior tilt | (C) Anterior tilt |

In general, the pelvic range of neutral is from 2 to 10 degrees anterior, and from 0 to 10 degrees posterior. But this is only an approximate guideline. We must not view the pelvis in isolation, but in relation to the whole body.

Notation of pelvic tilt

Notate the tilt of the pelvis in these photos by drawing a line from the ASIS to the PSIS, and from the pubic symphysis to the sacral/coccyx junction.

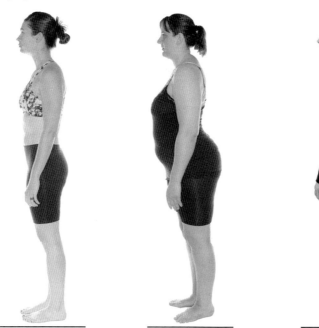

We now can transfer these diagonal lines to the body chart to notate the angle of the pelvic tilt.

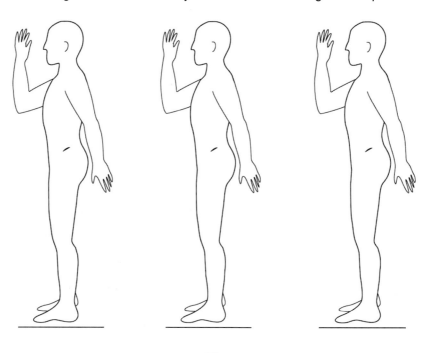

Tilt of pelvis/hip to placement with plumb line

The placement/position of the pelvis can combine with different tilts in many possible configurations. For example, the following figure shows that the placement of pelvis **A** and **B** is anterior to the plumb line. As you can see, however, the lift and angle of the pelvic tilt is different in each case.

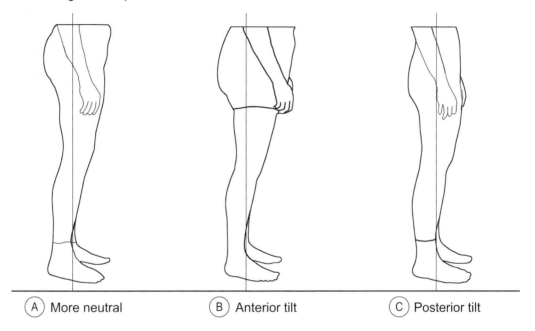

(A) More neutral   (B) Anterior tilt   (C) Posterior tilt

Study the following examples, which indicate other possible combinations. Also, note the distance of the ischial tuberosity to the femur. Often it's the lines of clothing (shorts, skirts) that quickly give you the information.

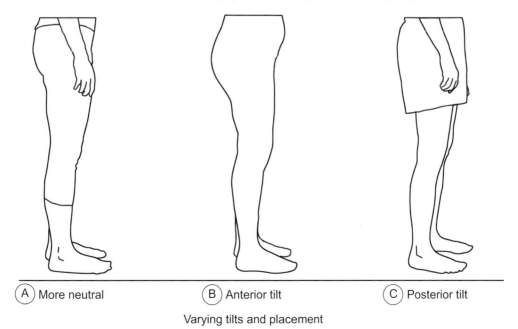

(A) More neutral   (B) Anterior tilt   (C) Posterior tilt

Varying tilts and placement

79

Varying tilts and placement

Exercise 5.7

Outline the segments on a transparency, then notate placement of the pelvis and leg, as well as the pelvic tilt.

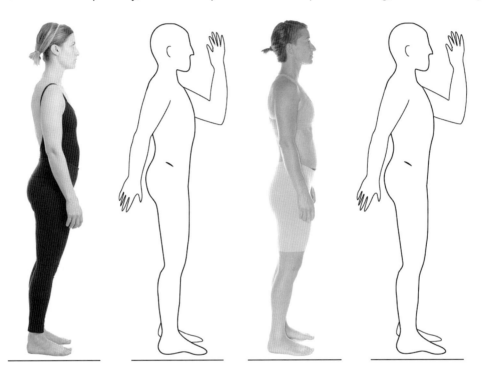

Remember that the X notates your reference point. An X under the ankle notates whether the hip joint is anterior or posterior to the ankle. Mark the combined placement and tilt on the body chart.

Implications

As you can see, the possibilities for the combinations of placement, shifts and tilts are many. This becomes important in determining how to suggest a modification to the client. For example, a common correction given to a person with an anteriorly tilted pelvis is to 'tuck the pelvis under'. If a client has an anteriorly tilted pelvis that is anteriorly placed, he or she may not be able to do this successfully, without first bringing his or her pelvis to a more neutral alignment. You may want to try this example with your own body.

Conversely, a person with a posteriorly placed pelvis, a posterior tilt, and a decreased lumbar curve may not be able to normalize that curve without adjusting both the tilt and the placement of the pelvis first.

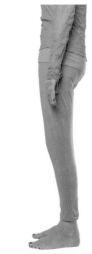

'Suck-and-tuck' pattern

Exercise 5.8

Notate the following landmarks. Upon completing each view, pause, and think about what your focus is from that one view.

Guide for landmarks

Front view: left to right tilts at joints

1) Top of head
2) Maxilla
3) Mandible (inferior border)
4) Top of clavicle
5) Shoulder joint
6) 6th rib to inferior sternum
7) Costal arch
8) Elbow joint
9) Iliac crest
10) Wrist joint
11) Hip joint
12) Tips of fingers
13) Knee joint
14) Ankle joint

Back view: left to right tilts at joints

1) Top of head
2) Occipital ridge
3) C2
4) Top of scapula (C7)
5) Shoulder joint
6) Across T6/7
7) Across T10/11
8) Elbow joint
9) Iliac crest
10) Wrist joint
11) Hip joint
12) Tips of fingers
13) Knee joint
14) Ankle joint

Side view: anterior to posterior tilts at joints

1) Maxilla to occipital ridge
2) Mandible (inferior border) to C2
3) Sternal notch to C7
4) Inferior sternum to T6/7
5) Costal arch to T10/11
6) ASIS to PSIS
7) Pubic symphysis to sacral/coccyx juncture
8) Knee joint
9) Ankle joint

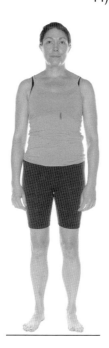 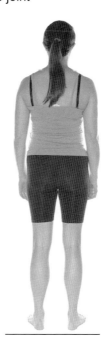 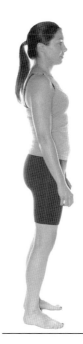

Now that you have notated all three views, which view gives you the most information and why?

Exercise 5.9

Practice by notating each view.

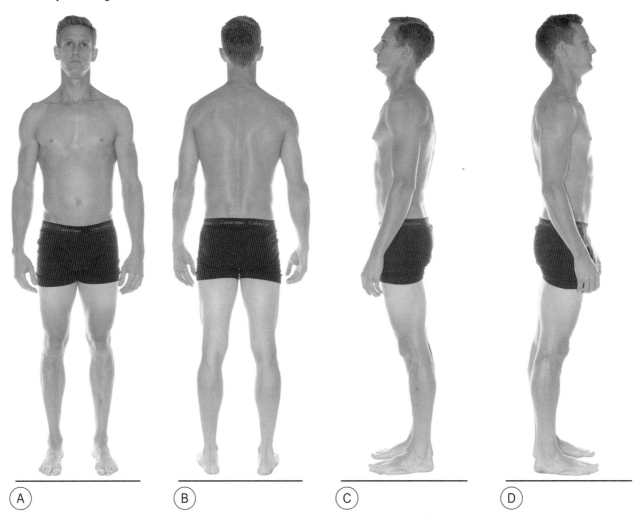

A   B   C   D

Which view gives you the most information?

I want to draw your attention to the different angles of the pelvis, as it sits on his leg, in **C** to **D.**

1)   In view **C:** ischial tuberosities are more down, behind femur.

2)   In view **D:** ischial tuberosities are more up or at a more neutral angle to the pelvis.

Remember that we are not just looking at one body segment in isolation but the whole-body pattern.

Pelvic tilt on right and left sides

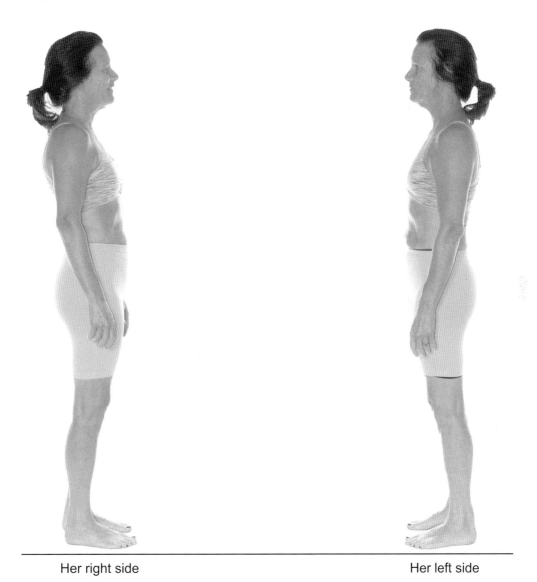

Her right side   Her left side

Compare this woman's two sides. Do they appear similar? How are they different?

CHAPTER 6

Up to this point, we have been emphasizing one plane of alignment at a time. Within each plane, it is important to view the body from both sides in order to get a more accurate perspective. Consider the two side views of the client below. Mark the centers of mass, connect the centers, and mark the plumb lines. What differences do you see here?

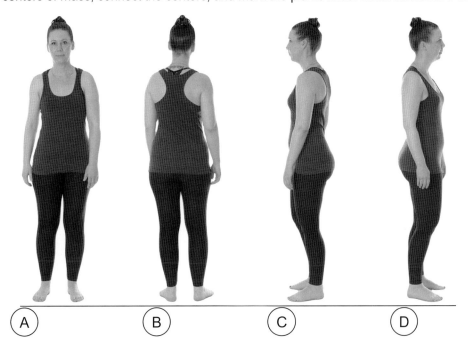

In comparing the two sides of the body, we clearly see that often their alignment is not the same, right to left. To answer how this can happen, we need to view all perspectives and the client's history and interests.

In addition to being displaced with shifts and tilts, body segments can also be rotated. As we have seen in the previous figures, a rotation can, for example, place one shoulder on the plumb line while the other is considerably posterior. The pelvis can be placed centrally on one side and forward of the plumb line on the other. Or you can see the rotation go all the way around that body segment, such as if the pelvis rotates forward on the left, back on the right, etc. I use the term *right to left anterior rotation* to describe a certain segment rotating forward on the right, turning toward the left. The rotation can be for the whole segment or portions of that segment, such as shoulder internally rotated, forearm externally rotated, hand pronated.

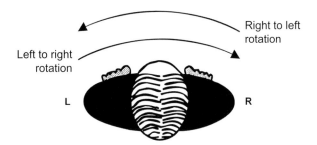

Look at **C** and **D** again. Observe the rotation of her arms, from right and left side views. Can you see that in **C**, her left shoulder and chest rotate forward, yet you can see her right leg is forward from this same view? Can you see that in **D** also? Now, observe how this pattern reveals itself clearly, from the front and back views.

Notation of rotation – 1

The process of notating alignment is the same, in the front and back views. Straight arrows indicate displacement of individual segments to the right or the left. Curved arrows notate anterior/posterior rotation, as well as internal/ external rotation of extremities.

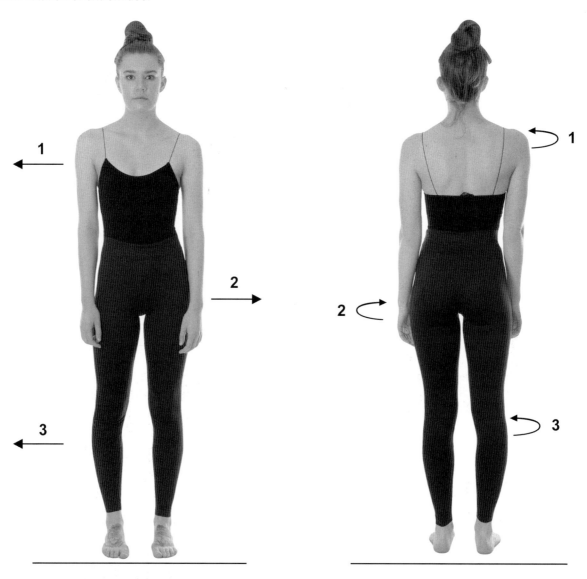

Rotations in the frontal plane

Exercise 6.1: identifying rotations

Mark the segmental centers directly on these drawings. Draw a plumb line and notice the relationships of the segments to the plumb line.

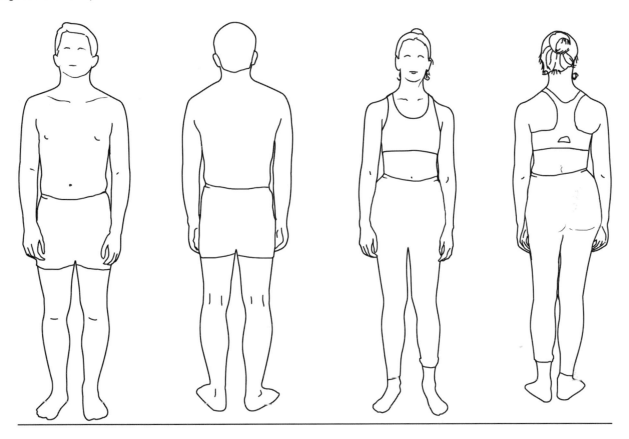

Do these segments appear shifted to the right or left only? Or, can you see the right or left side rotating forward or backward as well?

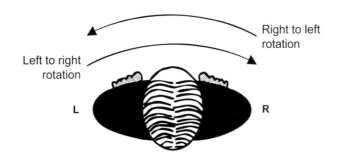

Right to left rotation

Left to right rotation

L   R

Notating lower extremity patterns

Once you identify the rotation from all four views, you can notate one segment, or several segments, as shown below. Vertical lines indicate the segment(s) being notated, with crossbars placed at the affected joints. Curved arrows indicate the direction of rotation: forward/internal or back/external.

A. The notation for one segment rotating internally or externally.
Example: Pelvis is rotated to the left.
Lower leg is rotated externally on the right.

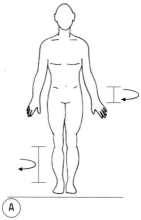

B. The notation for several segments that are rotated forward.
Example: The upper leg, lower leg and foot are all rotated internally.

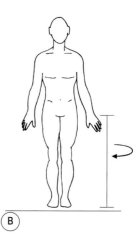

C. If the joint is rotated internally or externally, place the curved arrow at the joint.
Example: The left hip is internally rotated.
The right knee is externally rotated.

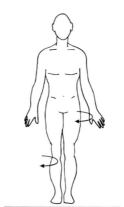

D. Combination: the notation for several segments rotated internally and externally.
Example: The right hip and knee are internally rotated, the ankle is externally rotated.

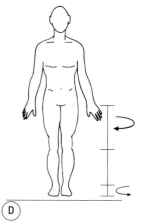

E. Combination: left hip internally rotated, left knee to foot externally rotated.

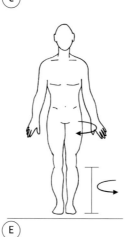

From the front view, we describe rotations as occurring from right to left (which means the right side rotates forward, toward the left side) or left to right (left side rotates forward, toward right). I am including the front view here, to show what can also be noted from the front or back. Observe the rotations in the following examples.

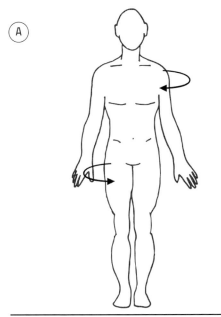

Right hip rotating forward (right to left) and left shoulder rotating forward (left to right)

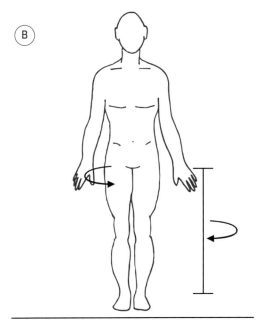

Left leg rotating forward (internally rotating) and right hip rotating forward

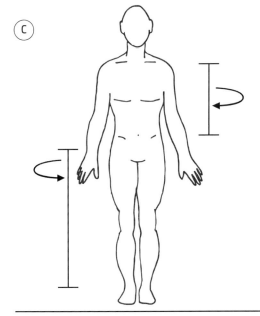

Forward rotation from hip to foot on the right side (R-L), left side rotating forward (L-R), from waist to shoulder

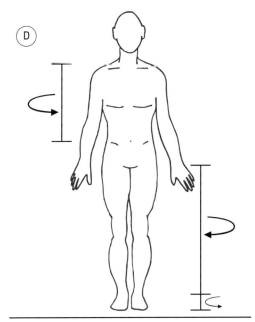

Left foot rotating out, left hip and leg rotating in, counter-rotation of right side rotating forward, from waist to shoulder

89

Counter-rotations

We begin to see that the body generally does not have one part in rotation, without also having other rotations. Just as a particular pattern often includes displacement forward and backward of the plumb line, it often has rotations in one direction and the opposite direction. Look at the examples of counter-rotations below.

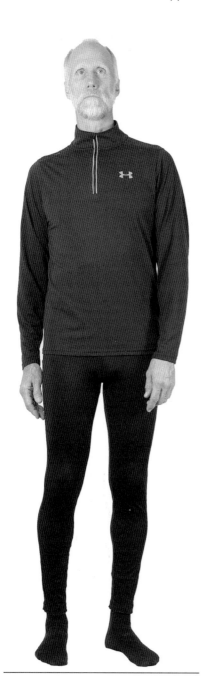

Left to right rotation at shoulder.

Right to left rotations at pelvis and internal rotation of right leg.

As you will see later, there are many possible combinations of rotations and counter-rotations. We will look at combinations in more detail in Chapter 9, to see the effect of these rotations in creating overall balance.

Example

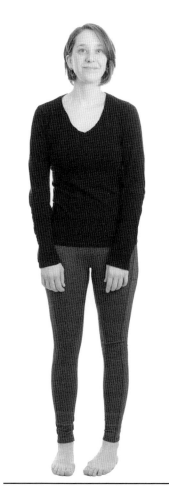 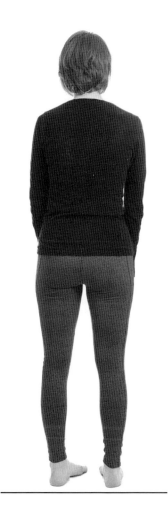 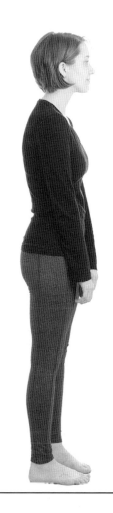

You have a sense that this client's lower body rotates forward on the left and back on the right. Also, her left leg is rotating internally. That rotation is also apparent in the side view, where her left leg is forward of her right leg.

From the front view it is not easy to see the counter-rotations of the pelvis rotating right and her upper chest and arm rotating left.

(Hint: If her waist area were also rotating forward on the left, you would not have seen the space between her right arm and body.)

Exercise 6.2

Draw geometric centers on the following three photos and determine whether there is simple displacement or rotation for each segment, by comparing the front and back views.

Note that, in this case, if the amount of displacement of a segment can be seen from the front and is also obvious in the side view, this indicates the whole segment is shifted or rotated forward or backward.

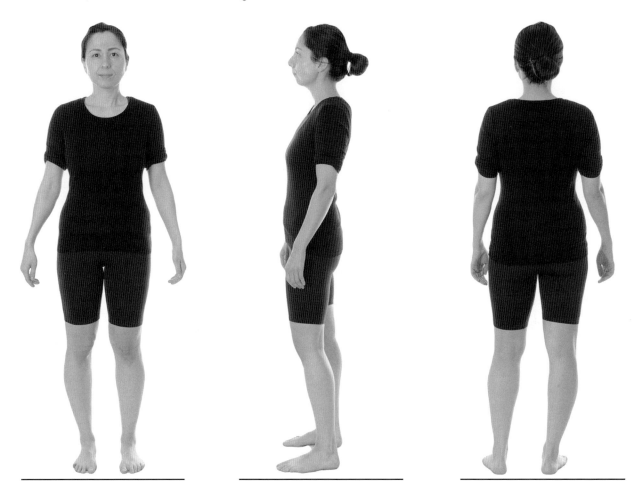

This client's right leg is more hyperextended and both legs are internally rotated.

You can see her counter-rotations:

- Her left leg is rotating forward left to right.
- Her pelvis is rotating forward right to left, which continues up through her shoulders, right to left.

Notation of rotation – 2

In order to document rotations, curved arrows are visually clear and can be used to distinguish rotations from simple displacements. Consider the following examples.

The curved arrow forward indicates that a specific segment is rotated forward or back, in relation to the plumb line.

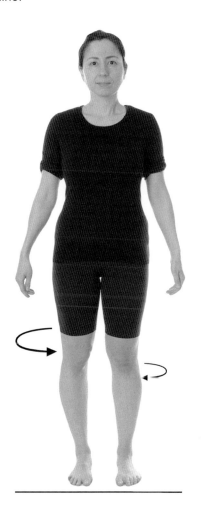
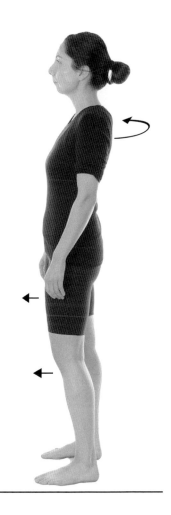
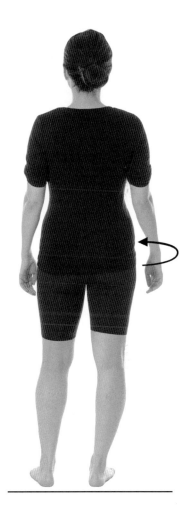

Exercise 6.3

Mark the placement and rotations for all four views of clients **A** and **B**.

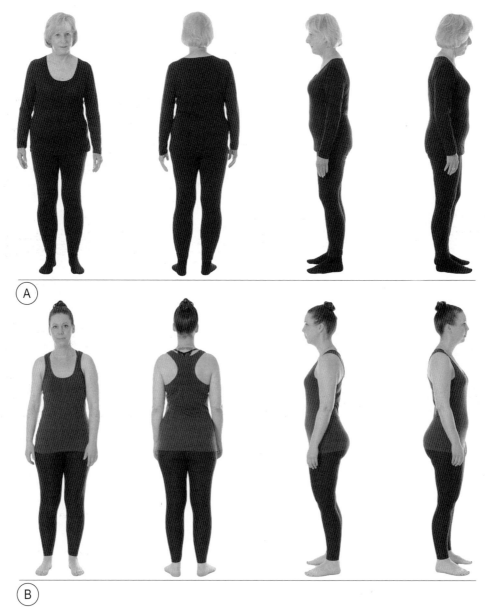

A

B

Interestingly, when looking at client **B**'s pattern from the front view, you can see that her pelvis shifted to her right with some right to left rotation as well. But that rotation is not as obvious when you look at the other three views. This implies the shift is greater than the rotation pattern.

For your practice and study, collect several sets of photos with all four views: the front, back, right and left sides. You may find it interesting to work with photos of yourself, as well as those of clients and friends.

Observe the following photos. Without using a transparency or making notations, observe which view draws your attention first. Then, which segment? Then ask: 'This segment is in relationship to which other segment?' Do you see more displacement, rotation or both?

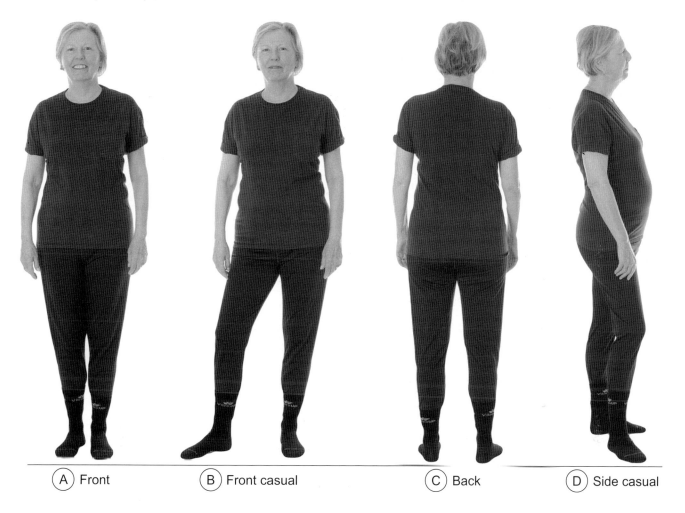

(A) Front   (B) Front casual   (C) Back   (D) Side casual

By observing a person's casual stance, you can often see how that configuration may neutralize some aspects.

For example, in view **B**, you can see the client's tilts at shoulder and pelvis are more level, compared with **A** and **C**. She may feel less tight or more comfortable in her casual stance. However, sometimes the adaptation of the casual stance is strong enough to encourage further compensation and asymmetry.

Legs – describing placement and rotation of the lower extremities

There are four basic placement positions of the legs:

1) Adduction–abduction
2) Anterior–posterior (flexion or extension)
3) Internal rotation–external rotation
4) Combinations

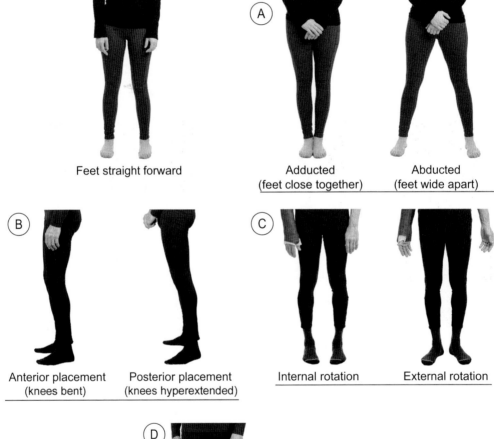

Feet straight forward

(A) Adducted
(feet close together)

Abducted
(feet wide apart)

(B) Anterior placement
(knees bent)

Posterior placement
(knees hyperextended)

(C) Internal rotation

External rotation

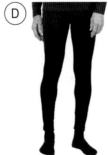

(D) Combination of the above:

right foot – slight external rotation
right lower leg – internal rotation
right upper leg – internal rotation

left foot – external rotation
left lower leg – external rotation
left upper leg – slight external rotation

Commonly, an injury or fall can result in segment(s) being pushed out of alignment. The segment changes position (is out of balance), and then the body finds a way to compensate for its new position with counterbalance.

Lower extremity patterns

People can adopt certain standing positions out of habit, because of physical need, or sometimes they stand in a way that they have been told is good for them.

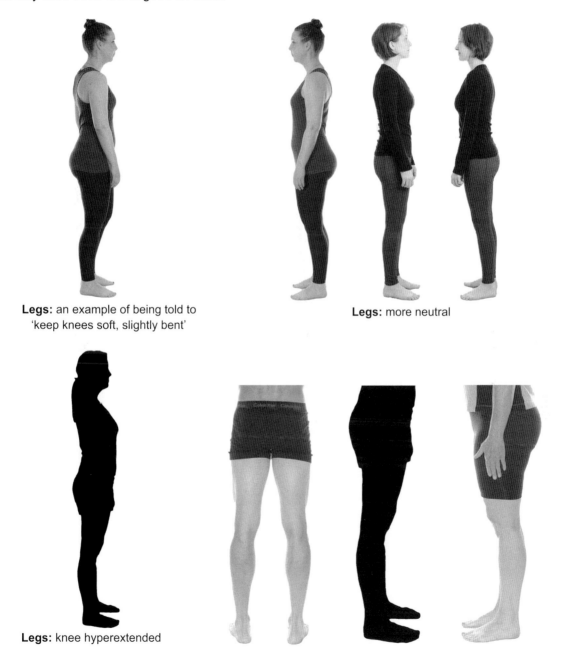

Legs: an example of being told to 'keep knees soft, slightly bent'

Legs: more neutral

Legs: knee hyperextended

Although these four pairs of legs are displaced posteriorly, observe the differences; because of internal rotation, external rotation and degree of knee hyperextension.

Exercise 6.4

Assessing patterns of lower extremities
A. Observe

1) The relationship of one leg to the other leg:
    - Tilt placement (high/low)
    - The front view – abduction/adduction (out from or in toward the midline)
    - The side view – anterior or posterior placement (including flexion and extension)
    - Internal and external rotation at the joints (observed from the front and back view, as well as from the sides)
    - The amount and shape of the space between legs
    - Combinations of the above

2) The relationship of one segment to an adjoining segment (upper to lower leg, or upper to lower arm) for:
    - Abduction/adduction (out from or in toward the midline)
    - Anterior or posterior placement (including flexion and extension)
    - Internal and external rotation at the joints (observed from the front and back views as well as from the sides)
    - Tilt placement (high/low)
    - Combinations of the above

B. Notate

1) Notate each view below. Use arrows for placement of shifts, lines for tilts, curved arrows for rotations.

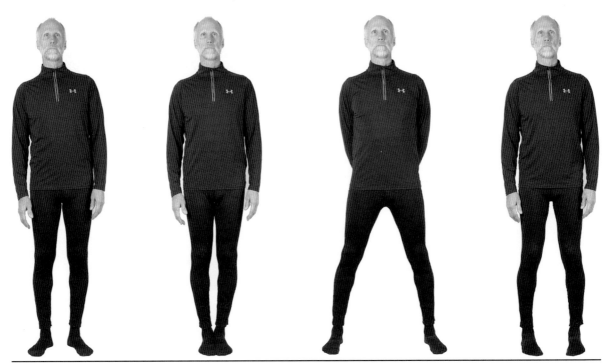

2) Notate the front and back views. Perhaps start by looking at the silhouette, to see what stands out to you. Use arrows for placement of shifts, lines for tilts, curved arrows for rotations.

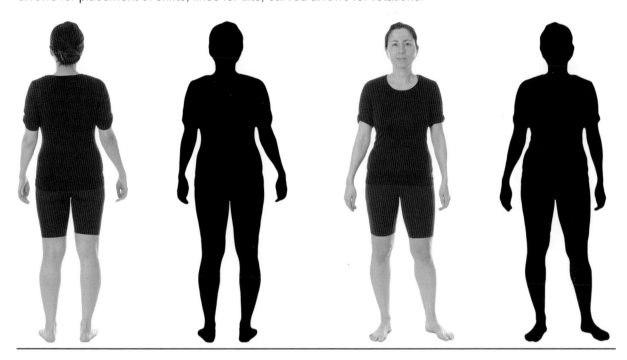

Exercise 6.5

Notate any rotations in the following patterns.

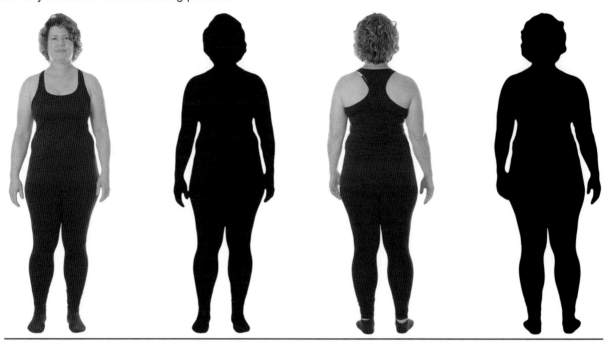

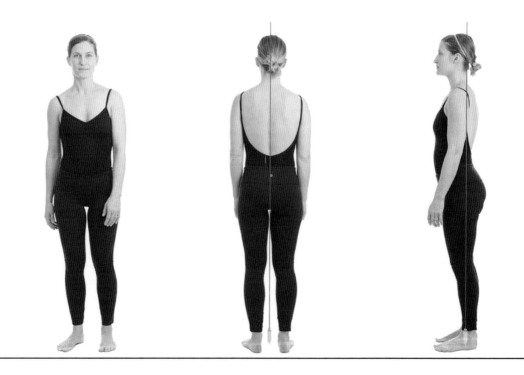

Exercise 6.6

You may want to use this earlier exercise of outlining the segments, marking the segmental centers, and connecting the centers as a reference before you add rotations.

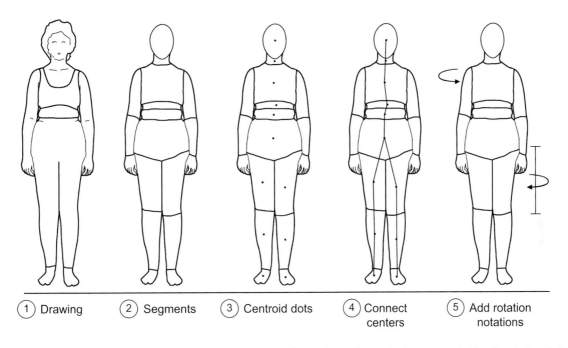

① Drawing ② Segments ③ Centroid dots ④ Connect centers ⑤ Add rotation notations

Now, look at the back view of this same person's pattern. Does it confirm what you see in the front view? If not, see if you can identify whether the different appearance is due to rotation.

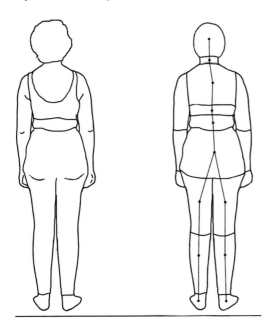

Note: The client is rotating forward on her left chest, which you can see from front and back views. But her upper chest is slightly shifted and rotated to the right, which is more obvious from the back.

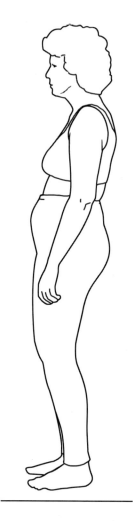

Observe this side view of the woman on the previous page.

From the front and back views, you were able to see shifts and rotations. From the side view, you may see the posterior shift, from her waist to her chest, and slight rotation of her right lower leg forward.

Let me draw your attention and preview another aspect that may prove revealing – that is *dimension*.

To get a sense of her natural proportion and the length of her body segments, look at her height from foot to knee, then knee to hip joint and then hip joint to waist. Now, compare the lengths of her lower body with the length between her waist and shoulder. The shortness (or perhaps, compression) of that area changes the *dimension* of the involved segments and might be significant in creating the pattern.

Dimension refers to the internal volume of any given body segment and will be discussed in Chapter 9.

Placement of the upper extremities

An easy way to begin assessing arm position is to look for the contrast between the contour of the trunk and arms and the space in between them.

The space between the arms and the body gives you further information about the alignment of the trunk. Sometimes one arm will appear closer to the body than the other. This might indicate a shift or rotation in the trunk.

For example, in the silhouette (**A**), notice the shape of the space between each arm and the trunk. The shapes are clearly different. What could create the difference?

Look at the following photos, with your focus on the size and shape of the space between the arms and the trunk. Note the information this gives you about the position or shift of the chest and/or pelvis.

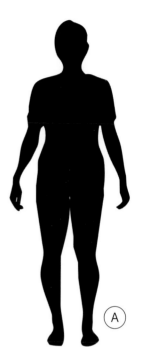

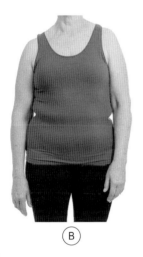
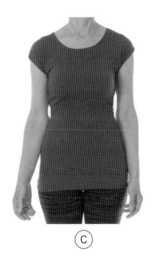
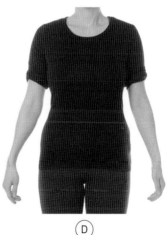

Exercise 6.7

Following the previous observation sequence, continue to check the placement of the segments.

1) The right to left (or side to side) relationship of segmental shifts.

2) The up to down, high to low tilts:

    B) Pelvis more right of chest, lower chest is shifted left of pelvis, upper chest is shifted right and tilted high on left

    C) Chest and pelvis shifted right

    D) Pelvis is shifted to the right of the plumb line and the chest is shifted to the left of the pelvis

Seeing rotations

The following are three of the arm's basic positions.

1) Abducted/adducted

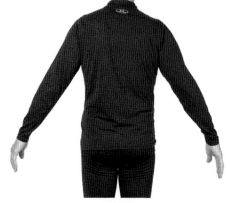
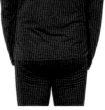

Abducted   Adducted

2) Anterior/posterior placement

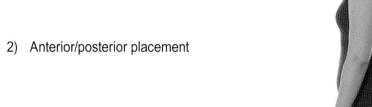

Anterior   Posterior

3) Internal/external rotation (pronation and supination of hand)

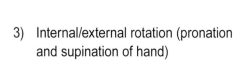
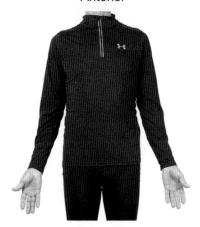
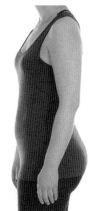
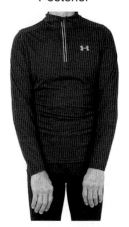

External rotation   Internal rotation

Combinations and notations

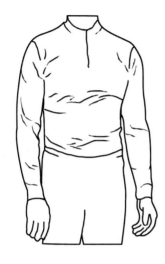

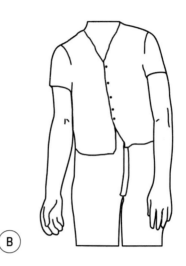

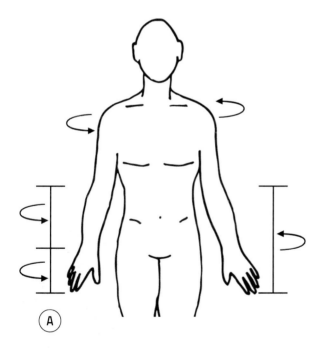

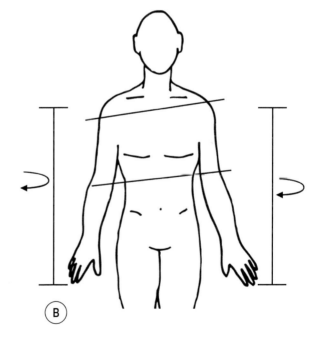

A

- Right shoulder forward, left shoulder back
- Right upper arm, lower arm and hand internally rotated
- Left arm externally rotated

B

- Tilt of chest/shoulder low right, higher left
- Right arm externally rotated
- Left arm internally rotated

105

Upper and lower extremity patterns

Describe the placement patterns on these sets of leg and arm patterns.

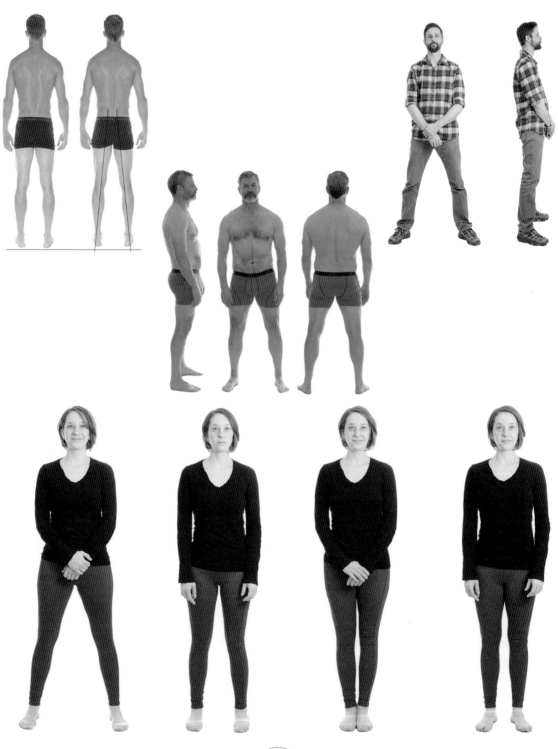

A. For the following figures, observe:

The relationship of one arm to the other or to the trunk, from the front.

1) Front: the amount and shape of space between the arm and trunk

2) Front: the transverse plane tilt – up to down placement

3) Front: the frontal plane – abduction/adduction (out from or in toward the midline)

4) Compare with the back view

5) Side: the sagittal plane – anterior or posterior placement of segment (including flexion and extension at the joints and hands)

6) Internal and external rotation at the joints (which can include pronation and supination of the forearms)

7) Combinations of the above

More specifically, look at the relationship of one segment to another, within the same arm (upper to lower arm or hand). There are many possible combinations, here are a few examples.

1) Is the shoulder internally or externally rotated?

2) Is the elbow rotated, in the same or opposite direction?

3) Is there flexion or a neutral position at the joints?

4) Does there seem to be a connection between the arm pattern and the uneven height of the shoulders?

B. Notate

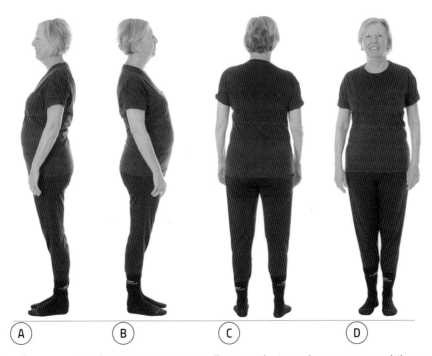

A   B   C   D

Check photo **A** again. Can you see the arm patterns easily, now that you have assessed the pattern from the other views?

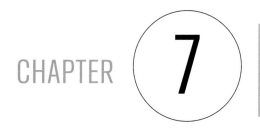

CHAPTER 7

Combining tracks

A track can be defined as a course of action, a progression, or a train of ideas. I apply the term *track* to the particular area of focus – shifts, tilts or rotations – which provides the most information about a body pattern. Can the same track be used throughout a body assessment? Sometimes another segment that tilts very much can't be found, or another segment that shifts to the right or left, and so we may need to change the track to define and summarize the body pattern.

As an example of having too many tracks, a client may have an anterior to posterior shift of the pelvis, and a strong tilt of the upper chest, compressed short in front and stretched long in back, as well as a shift of their chest to the left and a strong rotation pattern of the right leg.

These observations may be quite accurate, but synthesizing the information is difficult without feeling the need to neutralize every pattern. Often, we must step back to see another segment within the same track. We need to see if we can compare shifts to shifts, tilts to tilts, and rotations to rotations. Sometimes it will be obvious, for example, that two main tracks have our attention. At these moments we need to prioritize, to select the primary track and make the other our secondary track.

As you work, you may find that the first track changes quickly and makes the secondary track even more clear. This does not mean that you will necessarily need to address both tracks in that same session. The client may need to adjust to the changes from the primary track session for a few days, before more information and change is introduced.

Notation symbols

Here, we expand our group of notation symbols for various segmental placements.

Notations		
A: General Reference		
1. Reference point	✕	Starting from feet up, or starting from head down
2. Dot	•	Geometric center (centroid)
3. Line	●━━━●	Draw lines to connect centers
B: Placement/Shifts		
1. Right and left*	→ ←	*Looking at your client is a mirror image. Remember to mark *their* right or left, *not yours.*
2. Up and down	↑ ↓	
3. Anterior and posterior	→ ←	
4. Weight-bearing center	↑	
C: Tilts: High/Low		
1. Low to high	<	To mark up-to-down angle; from front, back or side views
2. High to low	<	
D: Rotations - combinations in three planes		
With the body facing forward: 1. To indicate one segment (rotating) forward on right 2. To indicate one segment (rotating) back on right		3. Or many segments rotated in the same direction forward on left

Observing, selecting and prioritizing visual assessment information

The previous chapters contain exercises detailing specific notations for your learning, but you can appreciate that putting all the necessary symbols on a chart would be prohibitive time-wise and overwhelming in terms of the amount of information.

Prioritizing information

You need to observe the body from all views, noting which view gives you the most information. Generally, this is the view (plane) that reveals the most extreme or obvious pattern to you. **To you** is the key, as another person might select a different track to describe the pattern.

Use the following list to draw your conclusions from the client photos below.

1) Identify the view that draws your attention.
2) Which segment within that view catches your attention the most?
3) What is the relationship of that segment to the segment directly above?
4) What is the relationship of that segment to the segment directly below?
5) What is the relationship of that segment to the plumb line?
6) Begin to imagine possible symptoms or complaints that this person might have.
7) Compare your thoughts with the client's interest or complaint.

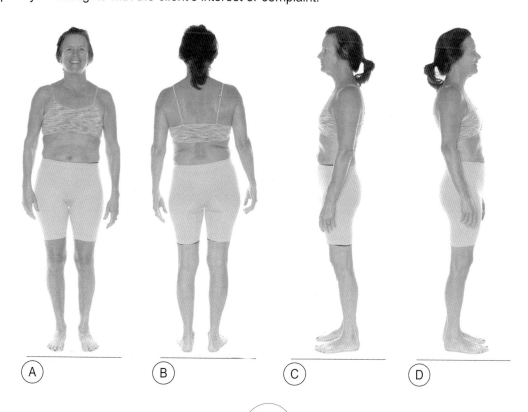

A   B   C   D

Combining tracks

Identifying and selecting the main track

As you begin to prioritize which view – which segment, in relationship to another segment – gives you the most information, you will select the appropriate symbols for your track:

1) Anterior to posterior placement shifts in side view

2) High to low (up to down) placement – tilts in side, front or back view

3) Right or left placement – shifts in front view

4) Rotations – combinations

As you identify which relationship gives you the most information, stay with that same track by comparing:

1) Rotation to rotation

2) Shifts (placement; displacement right with displacement left). Shift to right – where is the counter shift?

3) Tilts (right shoulder high to left shoulder low, and tilt (right hip low to left hip high))

For now, it will be useful to stay with one track, as you can easily confuse yourself by combining different tracks, such as making your focus:

1) Left hip joint rotates right

2) Shoulder tilt is high on the right

3) The chest is placed posterior to the plumb line and behind center of pelvis

When we have too many tracks in mind, it is challenging to assimilate them into a treatment plan. This is then confusing for you and the client. It is particularly challenging to resist the urge (either our own or the client's) to 'fix' all the observed patterns. This may be why we used to teach people to hold the line of posture, for their 'benefit'.

This technique will reveal if your selected areas of focus have a corresponding segment in the same track. For example, if you observe the whole chest rotates forward on the right and you do not see a counter-rotation in another segment, this may indicate that a different track will give you more information.

From a different view, you may see internal rotation of the right hip is the strongest pattern in relationship to the right shoulder's internal rotation, this may direct you to see how the left side contributes to the pattern. Perhaps the left side is tight and pushing the body to the right, making it internally rotate. Sometimes this is when your client reveals 'Oh, I did fall off my garage roof to the ground and landed on my left side'...and it all makes more sense.

Exercise 7.1

Now practice by notating each view.

1) Anterior to posterior placement shifts, in side views.
2) High to low (up to down) placement – tilts, in side, front or back views.
3) Right or left placement – shifts, in front and back views.
4) Rotations – combinations.
5) Choose a track.
6) Notate (refer to the symbol chart at the beginning of this chapter).
7) Upon viewing your notations, which view do you select as giving the most information?

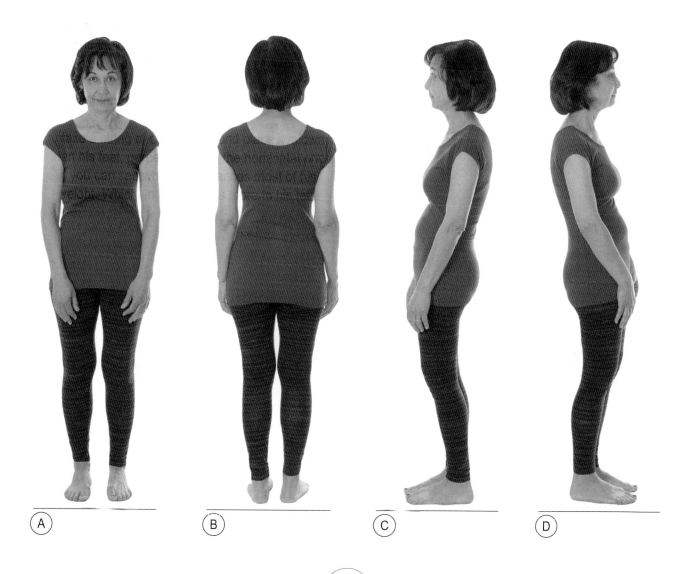

(A)　　　　(B)　　　　(C)　　　　(D)

Combining tracks

Notating upper extremity patterns

Notice in side view, that although the woman's right upper and lower chest are centered behind the plumb line, her arms are internally rotated at her shoulder and elbow, which brings her forearm forward (anterior).

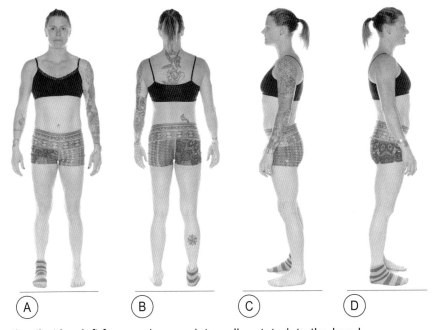

More specifically, notice that her left forearm is more internally rotated, to the hand.

In the front and back views, we could select from a few different tracks: displacement right and left, up to down, or rotation. As one example, let us select the rotation track. Some of the rotations would be notated as:

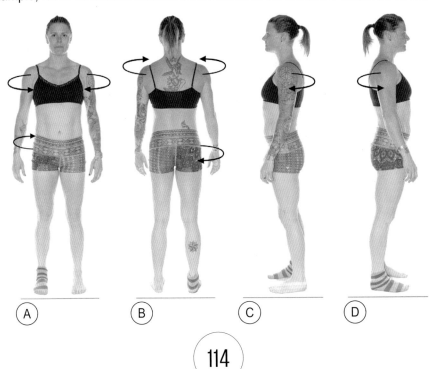

Notation combinations

The following examples indicate an easy way to notate the arm position. We are able to see the relationship of the arm to the plumb line, as well as the relationships between the segments of the arm.

In this example, we can see that the woman's arms at the shoulders and the forearms need to go forward and internally rotate, in order to counterbalance her chest displacement posteriorly.

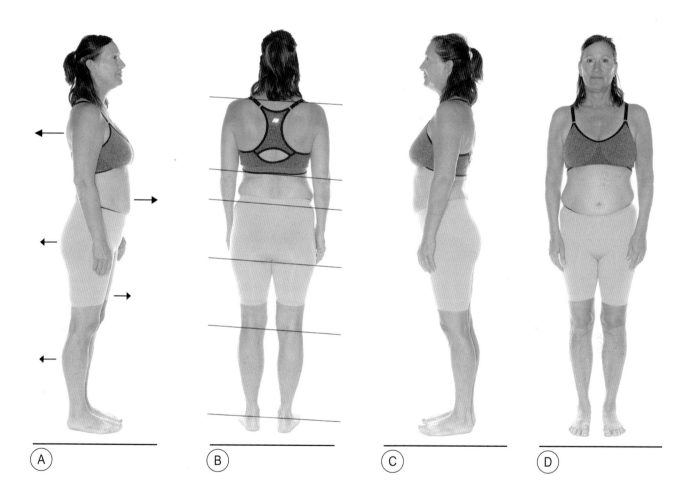

A   B   C   D

Exercise 7.2

Overall, this client's position looks good.

1) First, decide if you are starting your assessment from the feet up, or the head down.

2) Let's start at the feet. Take a blank piece of paper and cover the rest of the body above the feet.

3) Now slide the paper up slowly, so you see how the angle of the lower leg is placed. Is it straight (vertical) or leaning back (as in hyperextension at the knee) or is it leaning forward, to the knee?

   a) In this case, it slants anteriorly.

   b) With your paper still covering from the knee up, imagine what her body would look like if it were aligned directly up, in that same angle, all the way to her head.

   c) Take your dental floss starting from the middle of the ankle and follow the angle of her lower leg upward.

   d) You can see that if her body, from thigh to head, were in the same line with her ankle and lower leg, her whole body would angle forward by almost 10 degrees.

4) But as you slide the paper up, you see that her pelvis and chest are placed back (behind the center of her lower leg line). This is a counter balance to her legs leaning forward.

5) She has counterbalanced herself, by leaning her upper body back. Maybe because of demands on her body, from her work as a veterinarian.

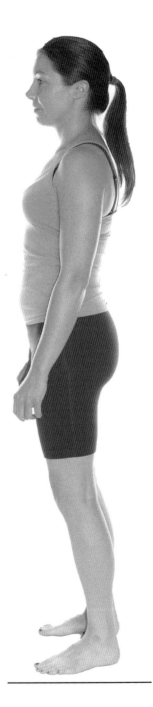

The body is always finding ways to negotiate restrictions to better center itself. When one part goes forward, another part often compensates by leaning back to balance. And so it goes, throughout the system.

Repeat the exercise from the previous page for clients **A**, **B** and **C**, below. Cover their patterns with a piece of paper and start either from the neck down or the ankle up.

A. If you started at the ankle, you would see that not only does the lower leg appear angled forward (like the previous client photo), but that the whole body actually stays in that same forward lean, all the way up.

This position does not show obvious counterbalances of segments leaning back. How does the client do this?

I happen to know (as she is 'posing' in this photo) that she can achieve and sustain this pattern by increasing ↑ her tension/effort through her legs and back muscles, to negotiate the amount of lean into gravity's pull.

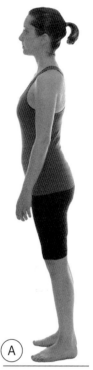

Ⓐ

B. Here is a good example of body segments progressively adjusting to the segment above or below.

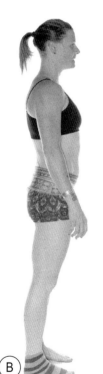

Ⓑ

Placement:

- Ankle to knee angles back
- At knee to thigh – forward
- At pelvis – back
- At abdomen – forward
- At chest – going back
- At neck – forward
- Head – centered on neck

Or, you could look at tilts:

Tilts:

- Just below knee – tilted low in front, high in back
- At hip/pelvis – slightly down and back
- At abdomen – tilted forward
- At chest – tilted back
- At neck – tilted slightly forward

C. Again, cover the body with your paper. Start at the ankle, revealing one segment at a time, as follows:

- To knee
- To hip
- To waist
- To lower ribs
- To upper ribs
- To neck
- To head

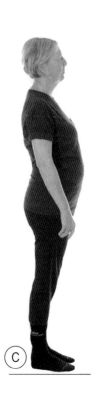

Ⓒ

As you look at the legs, up to the waist, you begin to have a sense of the client's body proportion. When you observe her chest (lower part forward, upper part back), you see that she has lost some of her body's proportion of length, from chest to head.

This example of displacement and compression can create more stress on a body and does not provide as much support as needed, for the neck and head.

Combining tracks

Observing a combination of tilts, shifts and placement, together.

Use paper to cover the body pattern. Starting from the feet up:

- the lower legs angle out;
- not as much at the hip joint, so there is probably additional effort needed, to negotiate the leg pattern to the hip;
- but at the waist, you see the pelvis tilts low on the right, high on the left;
- up to the band on the sports bra, the angle lessens;
- then the angle increases again, in the upper ribs, shoulder and neck.

This fits with the client's job as a right-handed hair stylist, who leans to the right most of the day.

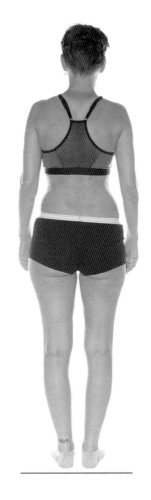

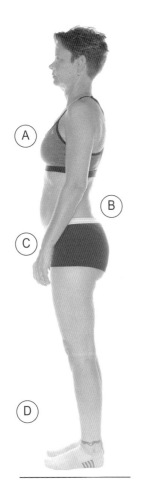

From the side view, the tilts reveal different negotiations with segments than the back view (above).

Draw the tilt angles for each segment in the side view.

1. Her lower ribs/bra line is high in front and lower in the back. 2. The top of her pelvis is high in back and lower in front. 3. Her lower leg angles high in back and low in front. 4. At the hip she looks more level until the knee.

Note: Watch for lines that would eventually cross (intersect). Where the tilt lines (if extended) would eventually intersect reveal areas of greater stress from compression. Opposite the compression side (where the tilt lines open wider) reveals areas of potential traction (if the segment is forced to stretch too long for its natural function). In this case, observe the segments labeled **A**, **B**, **C** and **D**. Do they look compressed on one side of the segment and stretched on the opposite side?

Mid-test

Look again at this photo, which you used for Pre-test A in Chapter 1. Note what you see, in terms of shifts, tilts and rotations.

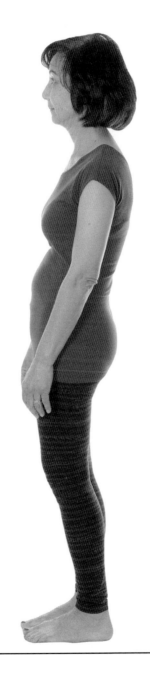

Are your observations the same? Are you gathering different information or seeing additional relationships?

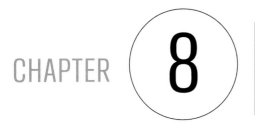

Introduction

From 1963 to 1974, I taught a more standard or familiar postural model. After years of experience, I began to correlate my observations and became intrigued that I had rarely seen:

1) The ideal posture in a standing position, being held without any effort.

2) A symmetrical alignment of the right and left sides of the body.

3) A symmetrical shape, where the dimensions of the right and left side of the body were the same – mirroring each other.

4) An even distribution of the body weight onto both feet, in the same way, and therefore creating an even wear pattern on the bottom of shoes.

5) The feet in a shape and position that supported the whole body above the foot.

6) The use of good posture, in a dynamic way, throughout motion.

I particularly witnessed this holding of so-called 'ideal' or 'good posture' when I taught movement education. It became obvious to me that, instead of my 20 students showing me there were 20 unique bodies in the room, they exemplified only one idea of the so-called ideal posture when instructed. I was struck by the loss of individuality.

As I began to explore postural models and their origins, I realized how 'ideal posture' had not only given people and their bodies 'rules' to hold on to, but also influenced the way fitness and rehabilitation exercises are taught, and how furniture, shoes and other products are designed.

Here are examples of my questions and realizations:

Question 1: Are the right and left sides of the body supposed to be a mirror image of each other, and if they are not, are we aberrated?
Realization: The asymmetry of the organs from one another in number, size, weight, shape, position and function, and the fact that we develop through these systems in utero, must set up a natural asymmetry in the body's right to left sides, front to back, and top to bottom.

Question 2: Are we supposed to hold the body still, in 'good posture', evenly controlled by the right and left sides?
Realization: What if we accept the idea that our bodies are not supposed to be symmetrical? Perhaps the asymmetry serves a purpose of keeping the body in continuous motion, thereby rehydrating tissues in continuous response to gravity. Perhaps we have been stifling the body's movement and need to learn to use motion to our advantage.

Question 3: Is the body's 'good posture' determined by the alignment of the centers of the skeletal joints (ankle, knee, hip, shoulder and ear) in a straight line, directly over the lateral malleolus, perpendicular to the Earth?
Realization: This seems curious to me because the plumb line of this model, at 90 degrees up through all joints, centers the body weight over the back half of the foot. Why would we have a forefoot, if it were not needed for the specific use of support and balance? If that alignment model is correct, then perhaps we were supposed to have an aft foot as well, which would center the body's weight more evenly forward and back of the plumb line.

Question 4: Do we mainly observe and assess body landmarks to determine optimal posture and function?
Realization: I began to notice that people could be aligned with all of the joint centers on the plumb line, yet still not look in 'good posture'. I began to wonder about the role of shape or dimension. Perhaps the

combination of landmarks and internal volume of each body segment (shape and placement to the segment above and below) would give us more information.

Question 5: If you can see the body is in good alignment, in most of the joints, can you assume it can still be functioning at its best?

Realization: It is the ability to see, not only the alignment of body segments but also their shapes and dimensions, that provides much-needed information on function. It is the relationship of all these components with usage, that give us the most information.

The above thoughts created a challenge for me, as they posed a strong contrast to my previous learning. I realized that I had a solid theme to explore … I was looking for the best structural position that would encourage a fully proportional dynamic body function, as well as a functional model that would reinforce and improve the structure.

When I kept seeing the results of students and clients making efforts to hold 'good posture', I felt I had to persevere. I am glad I stayed the course, as the discoveries and benefits that came with a strong focus revealed a new paradigm…

The Aston Paradigm

The theories about the body's asymmetrical alignment and dimensions, plumb line use, etc., provide a different guideline for body posture. This perspective can influence the way the body stands, sits and works, in relationship to the forces of gravity and ground reaction force (GRF).

This structural guideline emerged from my observations, as well as feedback I received from clients, who reported feeling more balanced. This ease of balance resulted when no one body segment was borrowed from, compressed, or restricted by any other segment, in order to hold so-called good posture.

Many therapists have found the principles of this paradigm to be most helpful in working with their patients. Chapters 8, 9 and 10 include seven basic Aston Principles, for your learning and exploration.

Principle 1: Aston use of the plumb line

If you hold a string with a weight attached to the bottom, gravity will pull the string into a vertical straight line. The plumb line will be perpendicular to the Earth's (or floor's) surface. We often see good posture demonstrated by a 90-degree perpendicular relationship to the Earth. If you look at the weight distribution of the lateral malleolus as the center point to the heel, then equidistant to the front of the foot leaves most of the weight-bearing on the back half of the foot. Particularly when you also line up all the other joint centers over that point. This math contributes to the body often needing to stabilize itself to stay over that 0 point. In early years, I taught many students how to hold that line.

In standing balance, the foot is designed to be the greatest weight-bearing segment of the body. Centering the body over the *entire foot* in order to use its whole length creates the need to move the axis point forward – to the front of the ankle where the anterior tibia, fibula and talus create a hinge joint.

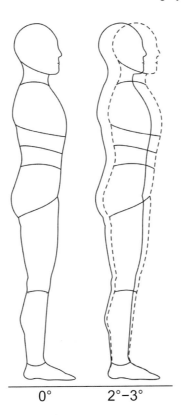

0°   2°–3°

Benefits of tilting forward

A) To negotiate the standing position, we suggest tilting the body forward at the ankle, by about 2–3 degrees as a guideline, to maximize the pull of gravity through all segments, for more even weight distribution on the whole foot.

This alignment also increases the ease of using the forces of gravity and GRF more directly through the spring-action arches of the foot, and the whole body. This poses a contrast to the weight being centered more posteriorly on the foot, which can cause increased tension or compression by taking the weight out of the forefoot.

B) We encourage the body to be dynamic: with minimal range of motion as needed and continuously moving. Because the body is in motion there are many plumb lines that are crossed in that motion. It becomes a field of many plumb lines and allows the weight-bearing to be viewed not as a single point but as an area, a range.

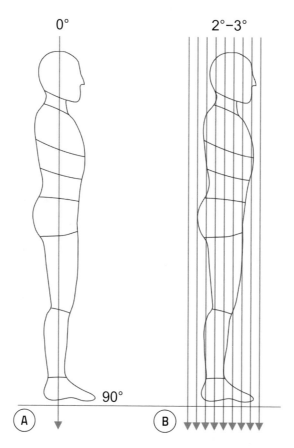

The moving central alignment line increases the use of the whole foot – its length, depth, width – which provides the fullest base of support (BOS).

C) If we pay attention, we can notice how every breath puts us into a new motion in response to the inhalation and exhalation phase. These micro movements enhance blood flow, exchange of nutrients, and joint lubrication, all of which are necessary for healthy tissue.

This dynamic posture encourages the body segments above the feet to negotiate the constant changes in position as well. The motion can provide moment to moment negotiation to the micro movement of the feet (in standing, or pelvis and feet in sitting). This is also true when movements from the upper body can gently influence the lower body. Hopefully this awareness can decrease the amount of holding or tension the body might accumulate during a day.

There is no sky hook!

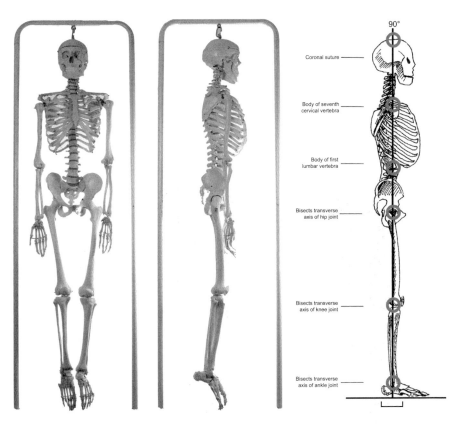

Perhaps you have seen a skeleton hanging on a frame in your anatomy class. And while our 90-degree skeleton (right) does look lined up in a straight line, when it comes to standing on Earth, this model centers the weight on the back half of the foot. (See the line, equidistant from heel to mid-foot.)

I started studying dance/ballet at age seven. It all made sense to me that I was being taught to lift up my body to be in good posture, and the image of 'reaching for the sky hook' was often the cue teachers used to get us in good position.

Then one day many years later, as I was teaching bodywork and movement therapists, I heard myself say 'But this image is completely opposite to the reality of the body on the Earth.'

We are not held by a string or a hook that would allow our legs to swing freely without weight or touching the ground. We are connected to the Earth through our feet, so the feet are weighted, and the head is free to move.

Suddenly it became clear why I had so many questions about the way people often initiated walking. They would start from a perpendicular position and extend the legs in front, to take a step. The resulting gait shifted the pelvis back and the foot in front, to pull the body along. I teach people to tilt the body first and allow the leg to swing under the body's center of gravity.

Initiating motion can be simple. You can start motion by leaning your body in one direction. You could take a breath, nod your head or move an arm – whatever micro movement allows you to gently put your body's weight into motion.

Principle 2: Aston neutral

Previously, I often started classes by asking students to demonstrate good posture. My students would show me good posture by trying to line up the centers of the joints: ankle, knee, hip, to shoulder and ear, into a straight line at 90 degrees to the Earth.

I was struck by how much holding seemed required to do this task and wondered if this much effort was needed to do so.

Dynamic neutral

My definition: 'Neutral is a specific configuration of alignment and dimension at any particular moment in time during which the body segments are in their "best available" relationship.' Neutral is not a point but a range that is a three-dimensionally balanced posture, and it is in continuous motion. This dynamic neutral offers stability and can balance the body from right to left, front to back and top to bottom. These three directions are combined to accommodate the internal structures, breath, and thoughts as well as the body's history of limitation, injuries and so on.

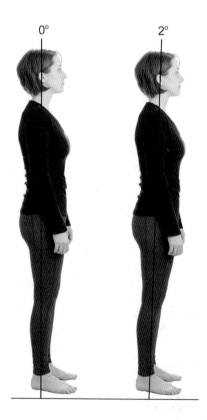

This neutral body is dynamic. It will sway up to 5 degrees, in all directions.

Neutral is when the body does its best to integrate all the history of influences (e.g., genetics, injury, sports, beliefs, personality, emotions) and finds a range of balance that is the least effortful. This neutral minimizes the need for any segments to overwork or restrict other segments.

Therefore, neutral does not look the same for everyone. It is a mathematical equation specific to each person and to each moment, because a mere thought (such as bad news) can change neutral posture.

There will always be an available 'neutral for any pattern'. Neutral is defined or determined by the person's pattern. It can be for the person who has an extremely flexed posture from osteoarthritis, or the person required to use a wheelchair, or the person with extreme scoliosis. They all have their available neutral.

We must factor in the greatest limitations. One patient might need to use crutches for six weeks, which means the two crutches plus the one foot (and the casted broken foot, off the floor) create three contact points to be used as the BOS. The best available neutral (without the cast) will be a different equation for three contact points. A stroke patient might not have much use of his or her right side. Another may be grieving over the loss of a loved one. There will always be a 'neutral for now' position that each person can find for whatever moment they are experiencing.

Base of Support (BOS) guidelines

The following structural guideline emerged from my observations, and the feedback I received from people who reported feeling more balanced. This ease of balance was achieved by increasing their BOS so that no one body segment was borrowed from, compressed or restricted by any other segment, in order to hold so-called good posture.

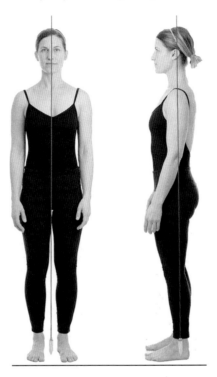

Front view

1) The angle of the leg is slightly externally rotated at the hip joint. This range may vary from 2–15 degrees outward for the feet.

2) The knees will appear to face forward but be angled slightly out, to match the open angle of the hips and feet.

3) The width of the foot placement aligns the heels (calcaneus) directly under the line of the ischial tuberosities and hip joint. It also aligns the forefoot under the line of the greater trochanters and the shoulder joint.

4) The shoulder joint is slightly externally rotated in order to match the forward lean and the external rotation of the hip joint.

5) The center of mass moves 2–5 degrees in all directions, in relation to the apex of the ankle hinge.

Side view

1) The central line of the body is inclined forward 2–5 degrees perpendicular to the floor.

2) The shoulder joint is aligned over the hip joint.

3) The body's forward incline of 2–5 degrees maintains the extension curves of the cervical and lumbar spine.

4) The head rests on the spine slightly angled forward and down 2+ degrees congruent with the lean of the body.

These references can be used as a guideline for seeing the body in stationary balance. However, because the body is always in motion and every body is unique, the reference point is used for comparison and is not intended to be a model imposed on every structure or person. In fact, some people will need to have a stance in which the legs are internally rotated to match an anteversion of a hip joint. This stance may be needed long term, or perhaps temporarily for overall balance until the person can be assisted toward continued change.

The position of the foot is consistent with the position of the hip and leg, which generally ranges from 5–15 degrees of external rotation. Please note that the angle is determined by the individual's current body options or restrictions; if a serious injury has occurred and the alignment organization is quite altered in order to match need, a person may need to use 0 degrees or 20 degrees of external rotation, with one or both feet.

Rationale: The open stance gives skeletal support to the depth and width of each of the body segments. The slight external rotation places the calcaneus in alignment with the ischial tuberosities and therefore gives osseous support to the body's midline. The position and angle of the forefoot supports the hip joint, shoulder joint and arms. Note, the height of the foot will be affected by overall placement and pronation or supination. Pronation tends to decrease the body's overall height whereas extreme supination can increase height, in a forced way that can strain the lower extremities.

Benefit: The position allows the weight and effort to be more evenly distributed throughout the skeleton and soft tissue. The joints are more evenly loaded, which maximizes optimal joint range of motion.

Because the two sides of the body are sometimes quite asymmetrical, they need an asymmetrical position of the feet in order to feel more comfortable and supported.

Position of feet

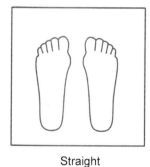 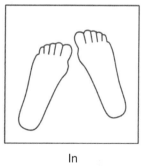 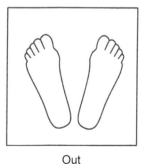 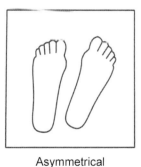

| Straight | In | Out | Asymmetrical |

When you look at these foot placement patterns, can you imagine possible leg patterns that might cause them?

If injury to the feet caused these patterns, how much would the legs have to adjust to accommodate them?

The motion available at the ankle and foot is determined by the lower extremity's joints and soft tissue pattern. Each leg is designed to support its own side of the body. If the placement of the foot is wider than the corresponding hip joint, it reduces the vertical support for the medial portion of that joint. Likewise, if the feet are placed too close together, the lateral portion of the hip joint has less support vertically.

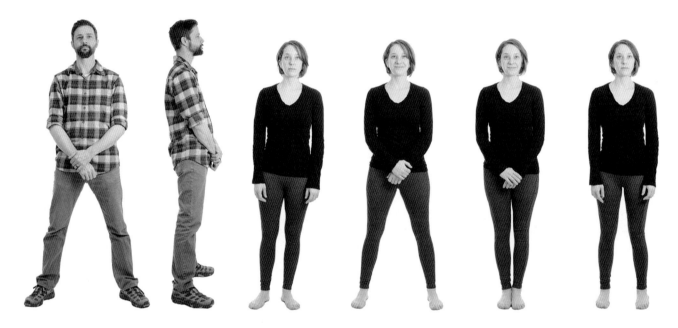

It is fine for someone to use a wide, narrow or uneven stance. It can become a problem if one of these is the go-to stance for most of the day.

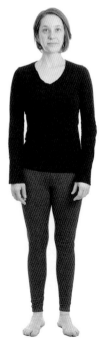

We find that a more optimal position is needed, to support the full width of each side of the body.

Therefore, the ball of the foot would be slightly turned out with the heels closer to the midline, to support the midline structures. The front of the foot is placed slightly wider to support the lateral line.

Principle 3: Range of Neutral (RON)

The body is dynamic

Traditionally, the main focus is that the body aligns itself around a central axis, which creates a specific midline of the body.

In the Aston Paradigm, even in stationary balance, the body continuously sways slightly to the right and left, forward and backward, up and down, in response to the gravitational and GRF forces. I call this dynamic balance the Range of Neutral (RON).

Because the body is continuously moving, the midline is a range across an area made up of six boney borders. The body sways between these six borders. The landmarks are:

Front view: from right side through to left side

1) Right side from the temporomandibular joint (TMJ) and costal cartilage down through the iliac ramus to mid arch of the foot.

2) Left side from the TMJ and costal cartilage down through the iliac ramus to mid arch of the foot.

Back view: from right side through to left side

3) Right side from the occipital condyle through the lateral aspect of the spine and sacroiliac (SI) joint to the calcaneus.

4) Left side from the occipital condyle through the lateral aspect of the spine and SI joint to the calcaneus.

Side view: back through to front

5) Posterior aspect from occipital condyle to posterior spine, SI joints, back of knee to calcaneus.

6) Anterior aspect of TMJ, to sternal notch, and pubic symphysis, to anterior border of the transverse arch.

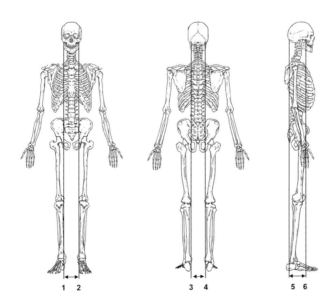

This position, even in stationary balance, is not static but dynamic. The range of motion (ROM) is 2–5 degrees in all planes. The guideline describes a possibility for optimum balance. Slight changes in degree also will change the amount of flexion/extension and internal/external rotation, as well as the forward/backward position of all segments.

Examples of RON

The Range of Neutral is determined by how far one needs to lean in order to feel balanced over one foot and then the other.

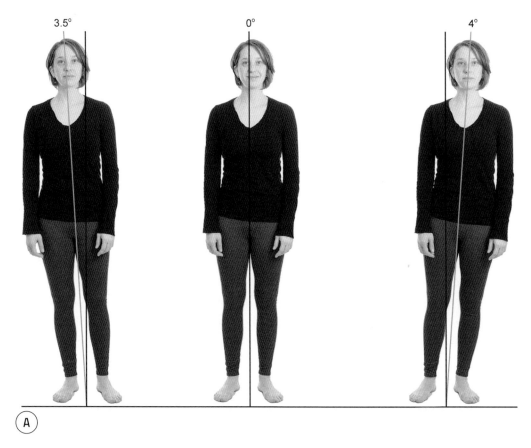

A

A. The woman pictured above has to move further to the left to balance over her left foot than she does to balance over her right foot.

Left image: her body's weight is centered over her right foot, leaning 3.5 degrees.
Center image: she feels centered between her feet, you can see she is still slightly shifted more to her left.
Right image: weight is centered on her left foot, leaning 4 degrees.

Note: the RON of 5–15 degrees can accommodate the unique body patterns of the male and female pelvis, as well as specific asymmetrical body patterns. Additionally, the two legs may need different degrees of rotation, including internal rotation, external rotation, abduction and adduction, in order to negotiate a limited range within segments.

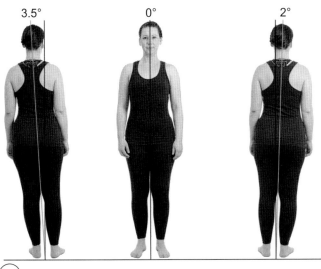

B

B. From the back, you can see this client shifts further to her left than to her right, to balance.

C. This client shifts further to her left than right, to balance.

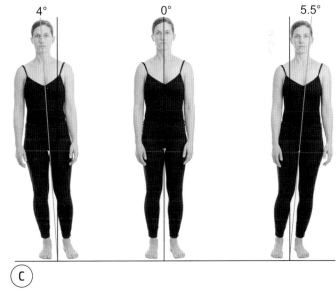

C

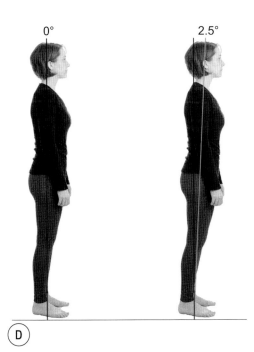

D

D. From the side view, RON will include hinging at the ankle and moving the body from 0–5 degrees, in all four directions.

Here, the client demonstrates feeling most balanced on her whole foot, titled forward at 2.5 degrees.

So far, we have been studying the placement or alignment of the body segments. Now let us observe the body's shape and dimension.

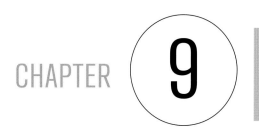

CHAPTER 9

Aston theory and concepts: Part 2

Principle 4: Dimensional integrity

History

My training in posture and body mechanics in college was always focused on lining up the body's joints (according to the standard plumb line) to be in conventional 'good posture'.

I remember being in Dr. Rolf's training sessions, listening to her expertise in anatomy, physiology, chemistry and physics. I certainly wished I had more of that knowledge. When she directed us to work with specific muscle groups, I became aware that I see bodies in terms of space, position and shape (dimension).

When part of the intestine or uterus is removed, for example, the vacated internal volume and loss of weight alter the body's alignment as well. When people have surgery to augment their chest or gluteal muscles, the additional volume and weight are also a strong influence on the body's balance. As I learned more, it became clear that alignment affects dimension and dimension affects alignment.

I remember when one big 'Aha!' moment happened in class. I was teaching my postural assessment class to Rolfing trainees. One of the practitioners was strongly placing his client into 'good posture', making sure all the joints lined up with the plumb line. The client looked quite uncomfortable holding this 'good posture', but kept up the struggle because it was 'good for him'.

His anterior chest was quite flexed down. I asked the practitioner if I could offer a few breathing exercises for the client. After a few minutes of exhaling out the holding pattern and letting new air fill his lungs, he looked more relaxed. As he continued the breathing, his chest filled out more anteriorly, in depth, width and length.

I then asked him to find a stance on his feet and to allow his chest to stay dynamic, with the breathing. We (the students and I) were able to see he was still lined up, but his chest was deeper to the front (the way it is anatomically designed to be) and his shoulder girdle was more neutral.

From then on, I emphasized this awareness of dimension in all my classes.

Dimension

Dimension refers to the internal volume of any given body segment and is one method of observing the body. The three dimensions for observing each segment (as well as the whole body) are length, depth and width. Together they comprise the available internal volume that gives us a sense of the space and optimal function within any segment.

This perspective of observing body dimension gives us very different information from that derived from looking at landmarks of the body. This view of the body includes observing the peripheral border (skin) to the opposite border of that segment (skin).

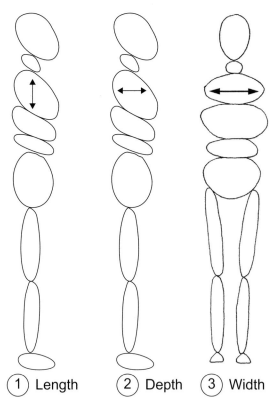

(1) Length   (2) Depth   (3) Width

1) Length: the vertical length; from the bottom of the foot to top of the head or the length of any isolated segment.

2) Depth: the horizontal depth; from the front surface of the body through to the back surface.

3) Width: the horizontal width; from right side surface through to left side surface.

When we begin to look for dimensional relationships between segments, we describe them in terms of a part being longer or shorter, wider or narrower, deeper or less deep, than another.

We can understand that in order for any joint, muscle or organ to function optimally, it requires the amount of space that is was designed to utilize. If dimension is diminished in length, width or depth, there may no longer be enough space for the body to operate optimally.

When body segments are compromised, a breakdown of tissues can result due to altered mechanics and disproportionate wear and tear. This can also set us up for decreased efficiency of the musculoskeletal system and the function of internal organs. For this reason, we can see that observing shape or dimension becomes an important tool for postural assessment.

Alignment to dimension

There is a certain amount of internal volume allotted to each segment of the body. When the alignment of one segment changes (the length, depth and width of that segment changes), it affects all other segments in some way.

Generally, when a segment is shifted in one direction, the length, depth and width increase in that same direction. For example, as one segment is shifted backward (posteriorly), the depth, length and width of that segment often increase in that direction.

When one segment (the upper chest) is displaced posteriorly:

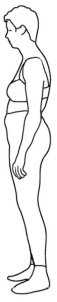

1)   The depth is increased posteriorly
     The depth is decreased anteriorly

2)   The length is increased posteriorly
     The length is decreased anteriorly

Looking at the front and back views, the upper chest is wider and longer in the front than in the back.

When one segment (the lower chest) is displaced anteriorly:

1)   The depth is increased anteriorly
     The depth is decreased posteriorly

2)   The length is increased anteriorly
     The length is decreased posteriorly

3)   The width is increased anteriorly
     The width is decreased posteriorly

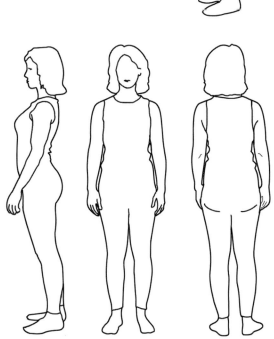

Example

In this example, the upper chest is centered more posteriorly to the lower chest, and the neck is placed more anteriorly to the upper chest's posterior position. Observe the relationship of dimension to this anterior–posterior displacement. How does displacement affect dimension?

1) Increased depth of neck, anteriorly.

2) Increased depth of upper chest, posteriorly.

3) Decreased depth of pelvis, posteriorly.

4) Increased depth of upper leg, anteriorly.

5) Increased depth of lower leg, posteriorly.

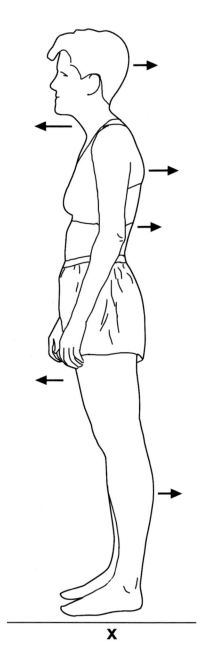

X

Flexion and extension patterns of the whole body

Although there are many possible balances and counterbalances within the body, I began to notice two basic patterns: flexion and extension. There are 12 components that make up each pattern. When you can identify all 12 components, you can quickly assess the client's body patterns.

To be able to see the many possible (and often subtle) combinations of the two patterns throughout the body, it is useful to identify and learn each pattern in its generic form first.

Flexion pattern

The generic flexion pattern occurs when the whole body moves into a position that matches and possibly exaggerates the spinal flexion curves that occur naturally, in the thoracic spine and sacrum.

Components:

1) Feet closer together, facing straight forward or internally rotated.

2) Body weight is centered posteriorly over the foot (heel).

3) Knees are flexed.

4) Upper and lower extremities are internally rotated.

5) Pelvis is tilted posteriorly.

6) Spine is flexed.

7) Breath is being exhaled.

8) Head and neck are flexed.

9) Eyes are gazing downward.

10) Scapulae will be spanned wide or can be protracted.

11) Body appears to be collapsing inward and downward into gravity.

12) Overall body length is decreased.

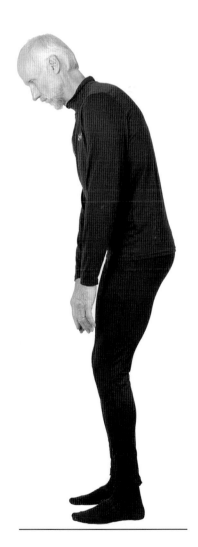

Extension pattern

The generic extension pattern occurs when the whole body moves into a position that matches and/or exaggerates the spinal extension curves of the cervical and lumbar regions.

Components:

1) Feet externally rotated.

2) Body weight is mostly centered over the forefoot.

3) Knees are between straight and hyperextended.

4) Upper and lower extremities are externally rotated.

5) Pelvis is tilted slightly anteriorly.

6) Spine is extended.

7) Breath is being inhaled.

8) Head and neck are extended up.

9) Eyes are gazing upward.

10) Scapulae can be retracted.

11) Body appears to be holding up, against the pull of gravity.

12) Overall body length is increased, anteriorly.

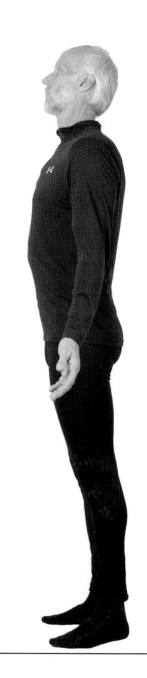

Practice with this pattern combination of consistent flexion and extension, until it becomes familiar. Then start noticing how bodies create variations on the flexion and extension locations, most likely in relation to their history and coping patterns.

Combinations of flexion and extension patterns

If body segments are in flexion and shifted more towards the back (posteriorly) the tendency will be more increased length, depth and width in that posterior position. Likewise, an extension pattern (the opposite) will move those segments forward, increasing length, depth and width to the front.

Where these two distinctly different patterns meet can create a stress area that is compacted all day long.

This body is mainly flexed, and the head and neck are extended forward and up.

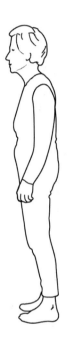

This whole body appears in an extension pattern, with the top of the neck and head in a flexion pattern.

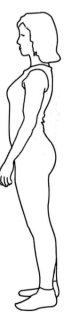

Combinations of flexion and extension

Observe the following patterns. How would you describe each person's body pattern? Can you see how the placement of body segments determine flexion, extension or neutral?

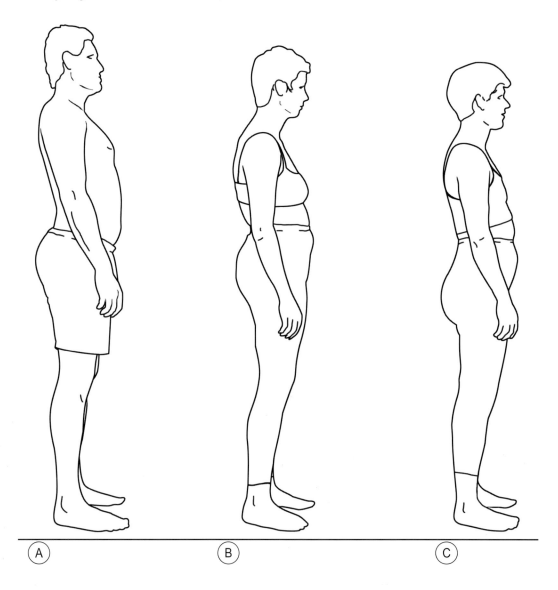

A · B · C

Would you describe client **A** to be mainly in extension?

Client **B** to have flexion at anterior chest and extension at low back, with compression?

Client **C** to have more of an extension pattern in the lower trunk and flexion pattern in the upper chest?

Observing and factoring dimension into one's plan can affect the sequence of treatment and exercise.

Exercise 9.1

Observe the tendency that, as one segment is displaced, this tends to increase the depth, length and width in the same direction. For each person below, notate the placement shifts that increase dimension in that same direction, then add the brackets to show dimension.

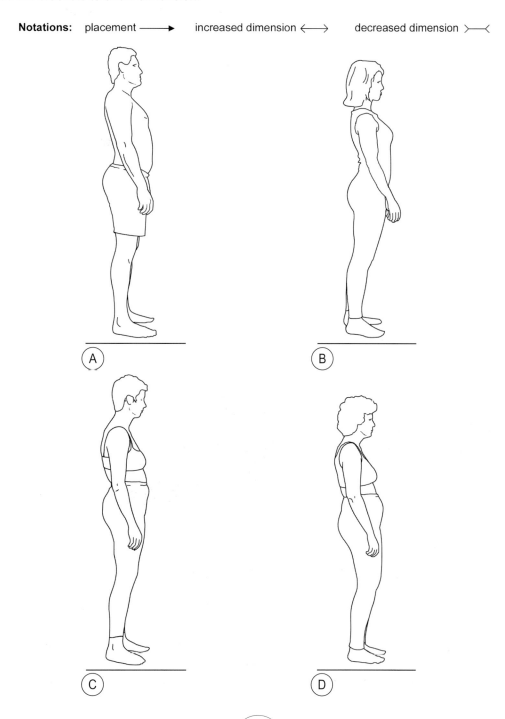

Aston theory and concepts: Part 2

The natural shape and volume of the body segments are obviously different in the anterior to posterior to lateral views.

A) Neutral chest

   1) Anterior view

   2) Posterior

   3) Lateral view

This pattern of the chest, with the person standing in his neutral position, displays a certain natural appearance and a matching of the chest's proportion from all angles.

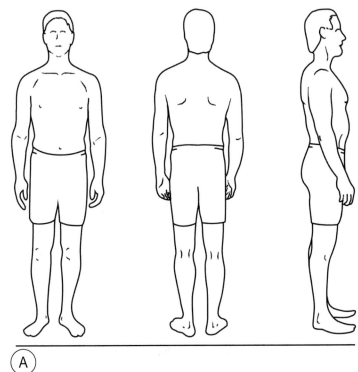

A

B) Flexion pattern in the chest

   Often, however, a quick glance at the frontal view of the client's upper chest reveals that it doesn't seem to match the size of the upper chest from the back view.

   1) Anterior (narrower)

   2) Posterior (wider)

   3) Lateral (upper chest, deeper posteriorly)

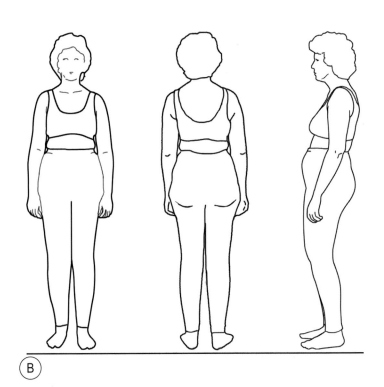

B

C) Extension pattern in the chest

1) Anterior – stretched out to be longer, wider and deeper than it is in neutral position

2) Posterior – in this case, the compensation reveals narrowing from scapulae to spine

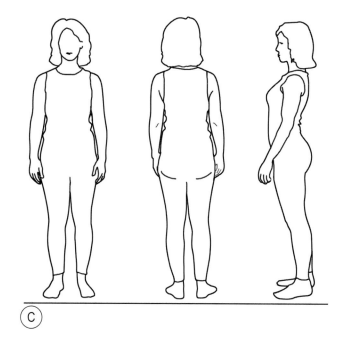

Ⓒ

It can be striking to see that sometimes the front view of a chest does not seem to match the back view of a chest. For example, the person may look like a much larger person from the back and yet the front chest looks very small by comparison.

The internal volume and function of body segments is determined by the available amount of its length, depth and width. For example, consider this pose of an opera singer finishing his aria. His posture may match the emotion of the piece. From the side, one can see that his lower leg is centered back to his foot and the upper leg is forward. The pelvis is forward and the upper chest is displaced back. In terms of dimension, his anterior chest is quite diminished in volume, which could affect his vital capacity for breath and voice.

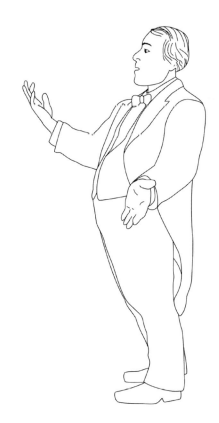

Notations for dimension

The following notations can be used to describe the change in depth, width and length.

Increased   Note the direction of arrowheads.

Decreased   Note the reversed direction of arrowheads.

Examples:

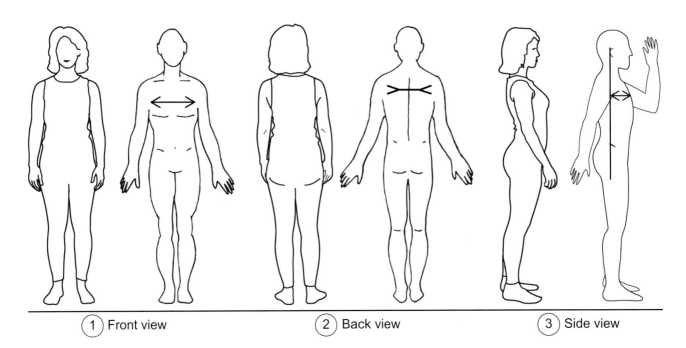

(1) Front view   (2) Back view   (3) Side view

1) Shows that the width of the anterior chest is wider compared with the back.

2) Shows that the width of the back is narrower compared with the anterior chest.

3) The client has trained herself to be deeper in the anterior chest, and less deep in the upper back of chest.

Seeing dimensional differences in segments

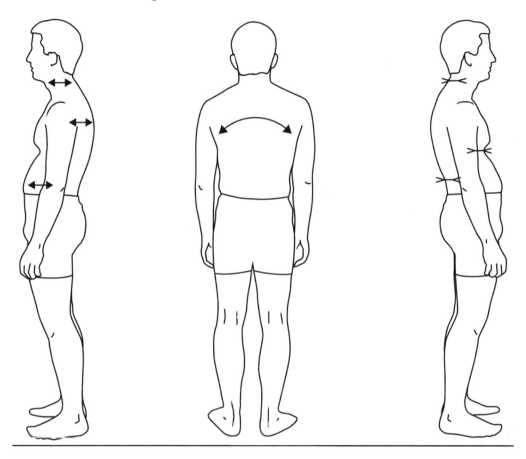

Example dimension:

- Front of neck deeper; back of neck, much less depth
- Back of chest deeper; front of chest, much less depth
- Front abdomen deeper anteriorly
- Lower back not as deep

Can you see how these increases in depth match the placement/shift of a segment, in the same direction? Posterior shift increases, but decreases the volume on the opposite side – back of neck or front of chest?

Tendencies of the body:

- As a body segment moves forward and back, it tends to increase in depth.
- If it also moves up, it increases in length and depth.
- If it also moves down, it compresses (decreases in length).

147

Example

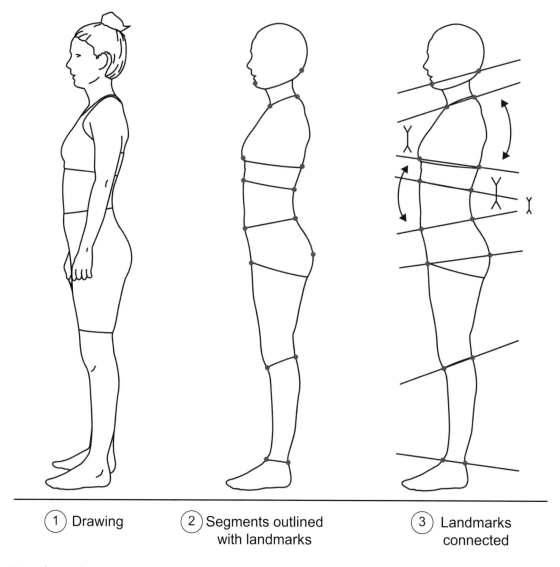

1. Drawing
2. Segments outlined with landmarks
3. Landmarks connected

Can you identify the flexion and extension patterns?

The area where the segmental angle changes direction can be called **a transition area**. These areas are examples of compression, shear, or torsion created by the placement, which could be the result of previous injury, usage or habit.

Remember, where lines demonstrate that they will eventually intersect are areas of shortness and potential stress. In the image above, **3** shows posterior compression between T10 and L1 posteriorly, and anterior compression between xiphoid and sternal notch.

If you observe the opposite side of the segment that is compressed, you will often see that segment is overstretched from its neutral position. See the notations for increased and decreased length dimension on the image **3** above.

Observe the combination of anterior to posterior placement with the up to down tilt relationship at the joints.

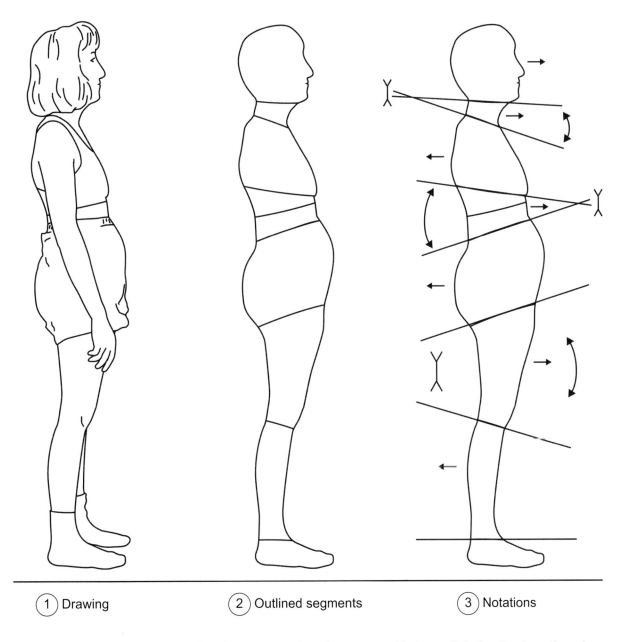

① Drawing   ② Outlined segments   ③ Notations

This combination of anterior to posterior placement and angles can provide immediate feedback on the primary areas of compromise. Each intersection of lines poses a strong possibility of compression, as well as the concern for body segment areas being pushed too long or deep, into an overstretched position.

149

Aston theory and concepts: Part 2

Alignment and aperture

Aperture is a term we use to describe the cross-sectional area of the body in any plane.

An example of an aperture would be any two-dimensional cross-section of a segment. These intersections of segments behave like the iris of the eye or the aperture of a camera. An aperture can increase, decrease or change shape, depending on its relationship to the adjacent segments.

The aperture can be observed in all three planes, to indicate the two-dimensional volume of any segment. For now, consider the aperture through the transverse plane (like an MRI scan) of a body segment.

When the body is in its more neutral alignment, the apertures are at their optimal functioning capacity for direct weight-bearing among the segments. The Earth forces find their pathway through the combined apertures.

The shape of the aperture will then be affected accordingly. Compression will often increase the diameter of the aperture, and distraction or tensile force can decrease the diameter of the aperture.

Now, let's look more specifically at how displacement, from one segment to another, affects the dimension and function of a specific aperture.

Observe the cross-section of the right thigh in this illustration. We can assume that this is an example of someone standing in the neutral position. Imagine how this cross-section would look if the person were standing in a flexion pattern, with weight-bearing over the right foot.

This would most likely increase the anterior dimension of the right thigh. The same components of muscle, bone and all soft tissue would likely be changed in position and dimension, by the biomechanical stresses.

Now, imagine the image of a person standing, with the pelvis and upper thigh pushed forward, the corresponding knee rotating internally, and the ankle and foot rotating externally, in opposition. How might this pattern affect the cross-sections at the joints? How might the aperture at the upper thigh change, from this amount of torsion?

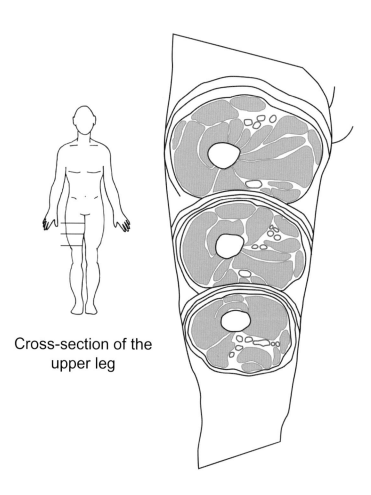

Cross-section of the
upper leg

Bird's eye view of placement and dimension

When a segment is displaced, the apertures of the segmental intersections will be reduced or expanded, according to the amount and direction of the displacement.

In the 1970s, I used to take my students to the mall for 'body watching'. One exercise I always included was standing on a second-story balcony, to observe another student standing beneath us, at ground level. I would have the students assess anterior to posterior placement and right to left placement of segments, then confirm their findings by observing from the front, back and side views from the ground level.

Two examples of this are in the overhead views of the body, below. Illustration **A** shows a more neutral position, while **B** demonstrates a body with several anterior and posterior displacements.

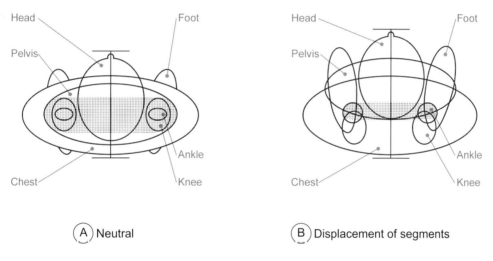

Ⓐ Neutral   Ⓑ Displacement of segments

A) More optimal weight-bearing from head to foot, throughout all segments. The shading shows direct congruent weight-bearing through all joints.

B) The shading shows minimal direct weight-bearing; passing only through the posterior head, anterior chest and posterior pelvis to the foot, with the consequence of less direct support for all segments.

Placement:
1) Knee posterior to ankle (note the tiny shaded area here)
2) Pelvis is forward
3) Chest is leaning far back

In gait, I believe there is a continuous sequence from one foot up that side that crosses over to the other foot and up that side and so on. The two sides interact through this cooperative and alternate spiraling.

4) Head is forward

From overhead, notice the vertical weight-bearing, where the segments intersect. This anterior to posterior and right to left displacement of segments reduces the surface area (or BOS), for direct weight-bearing. The shape of the aperture will then be affected accordingly.

Exercise 9.2

Observe the following illustration for displacement and change in dimension. Consider possible consequences such as shear, compression and torsion.

Review the aperture illustration (on the previous page) for this exercise.

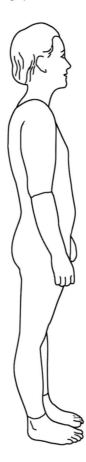

1) What track draws your attention first – dimension, placement or rotation?
2) Identify the other components within the track you choose.
3) Imagine outlining the body and placing the geometric centers.
4) Connect the lines in your mind. Check your visualization by using dental floss as a plumb line.
5) What are your conclusions?
6) Imagine this alignment pattern from the bird's eye view.
7) Now, as though you were looking from over the client's head, start with the feet and draw the segments (one on top of the other), with forward or back and right or left placement, according to your observations.
8) Shade in the body segment areas that are directly aligned in common.
9) What is your summary assessment?

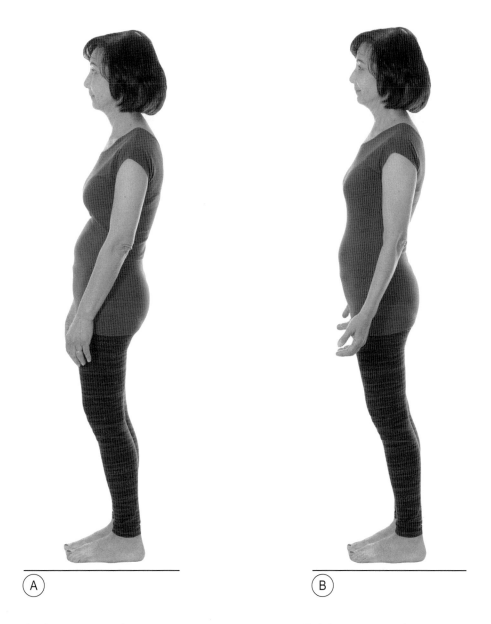

(A) (B)

Now, compare **A** (before treatment) to the more neutral position in **B** (after treatment).

How did this improvement, from **A** to **B**, change the weight-bearing of the client's segments?

When travelling in a car, we sometimes feel a jolt when the car goes over a speed bump. If we are sitting in a fairly good, aligned position, our body's shock absorbers work well to protect us. When the body is not aligned well, the impact from such an event can create a significant whiplash effect.

Imagine these two body patterns, sitting in a car and hitting a bump. Can you appreciate the different effect the bump might have on body pattern **A**, compared to body pattern **B**?

The three-dimensional foot

I emphasize the significance of the foot's three dimensions as support for the respective depth, width and height of the body and all its segments above.

1) Depth: when the foot is shorter than is optimal (from surgery, injury, shoes or usage patterns), it compromises support for the anterior to posterior depth of the body above.

2) Width: when the foot is placed in a wide or narrow stance or the foot has an inversion or eversion pattern, the optimal width is decreased, which decreases support for the width of the body above.

3) Height: when the foot is flat, pronated or has extreme arches or is supinated, it can influence and compromise the body's length or height.

People can learn how to optimize the best possible usage for their limitation, but often people do not know how to make self-corrections.

How did the feet get so far away from our attention? People often ignore their feet until there is a problem (bunions, strains, sprains, flat feet, ingrown nail, broken toe, etc.). I think the overall body design made the foot mathematically proportioned to support the entire body, above the feet. Yet the feet are often out of our consciousness.

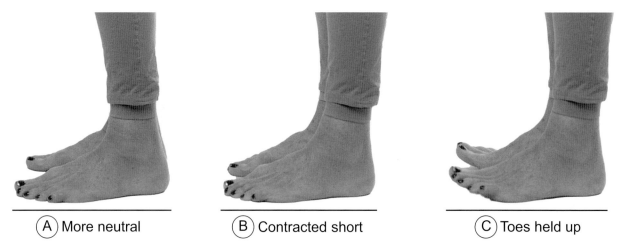

(A) More neutral (B) Contracted short (C) Toes held up

A) Standing comfortably, with my weight evenly distributed on my whole foot (having had many injuries and broken bones in my feet and legs, this is my best available neutral).

B) The foot is scrunched short, which decreases its overall length. For example, this could arise from wearing shoes that are too small, or from a pattern left over from an injury that impacted the toes on one foot, and which wasn't neutralized after the injury healed. How might this shortness affect the rest of the body?

C) I am extending my toes up which shortens the overall length of my foot, but also the top of my forefoot even more. I demonstrated this pattern because so many shoes are now designed in this way. The design is often justified because we flex the foot at this juncture, when we walk and run. However, this constant shortness of the shoe prevents us from using the whole length of the foot, to roll into and out of the flexion.

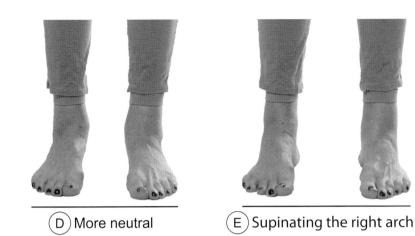
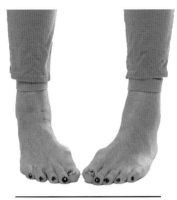

D) More neutral   E) Supinating the right arch   F) Internal rotation with inversion

D) Appears supportive to the structures above, however, with bone deformity, scar tissue and arthritis, the restrictions are felt more in larger motions than standing.

E) The supination of my right foot lifts and shifts my weight more over my left foot. This pattern also lessens the support for forward motion, as the supination pulls the foot out laterally.

F) More extreme inversion with internal rotation. This pattern can inhibit forward motion. Generally, people with this pattern have to engage more side to side motion, while moving forward.

Summary:

1) Optimally, weight-bearing can move directly through the entire foot and the foot becomes supportive to each segment above it.

2) In standing, the whole foot is used as a base of support. The right foot supports the right side of the body and the left foot supports the left side of the body. The front of the foot supports the wider and deeper structures above at the front, such as the chest and head. The posterior foot supports the back of the body.

3) Standing balance becomes a dynamic phenomenon energizing the body as its center moves to the right, the left, forward, back, up and down.

Principle 5: Asymmetry

Conventional models of posture often taught us to correct ourselves, so that the right and left sides of the body are more symmetrical. When I realized I had never seen this to be true in real life, I began to question why. I began to wonder if asymmetry was a necessary equation to encourage motion.

I have found there are **three main categories of asymmetry**:

1) **Natural asymmetries**

   - The congenital structural pattern. For example, the organs are quite different from one another in size, weight, placement, and functional influences. A person may be born without thumbs or missing one of the lobes of the lungs, or an extra vertebra, etc. These givens cannot be changed.

2) **True limitations**

   - Patterns that occur after birth, that arise as part of an injury or pathology and will be present for life. Examples might be a broken clavicle that healed in a compromised shape or a crushed right tibia that caused a 2-inch loss of bone and height in that leg. While our work, treatments, and lessons may facilitate relief, and clients can feel improvements, we cannot replace those 2 inches of lost bone. Thus, it is a true limitation. However, we might suggest an insert into the client's shoe or a lift added to the bottom of the shoe, to help balance and support the extreme asymmetry.

3) **Compensations**

   - Patterns that are not a result of natural causes, injury or pathology. Instead, they arise as adaptations to the other two types of asymmetry.
   - They can be the way a body has developed around the asymmetries, or by expression of emotional distress, or habitual use of their body's posture.

   - The good part of this third category is that it is the most available for change.
   - I have often seen people dealing with extreme variations between their two sides yet, when they receive bodywork, movement education and ergonomic consultation, the differences are often quite reduced; they feel significantly improved and hopeful.

The Asymmetry Principle is extremely important with respect to movement. In natural objects just as in the body, one observes asymmetry: within the strata of the Earth, the shape of shells, and the rings in the cross-section of a tree. Likewise, in movement, there are many asymmetrical and non-linear designs. Where the aspects of density, tempos, and direction interact, we see manifestations such as waves, a snowfall, and a flowing river moving in non-linear patterns. The body is the same. It is made up of a continuum of many different densities from fluids to solids.

The body also has many different tempos within the systems, in the functions of breathing, digestion and circulation. These, combined with our structural asymmetry, dictate that we also need to move in non-linear ways. I am not encouraging that anyone exaggerate asymmetry. I am proposing that, because of injuries, history or viscera, the body becomes asymmetrical.

Trying to contain all of these influences in right and left symmetry can create unnecessary holding patterns, negatively influencing the body's motion and function.

We need not be alarmed by slight asymmetries we see in the body. I think we have the ability to negotiate some asymmetrical differences. We merely need to teach the client to use each side (right and left) uniquely. Being able to *see* enables us to investigate what is a necessary or unnecessary asymmetrical pattern, for the many demands of action, activities of daily living (ADLs), sports, work and so on.

We want our homes and furniture to be secure and stable, not flexible like the human body. After a few years of secure stability we found the doors in our house no longer closed quite so precisely, almost as though they were off-center… Could it be the house settling? Or the Earth settling? Whatever the reason, asymmetries have revealed themselves.

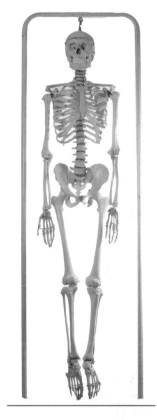

Even this skeleton has asymmetries. He has been hanging from his sky hook for more than 30 years now.

Notice how his right ilium rotates forward, which internally rotates and adducts his right leg, so we can see the space between his tibia and fibula distinctly. Gravity has taken a toll.

I am sure you all will have experienced the following scenario. A client presents with severe back pain. He is used to therapists diving into the area with both elbows. When you study his body pattern you see his pelvis is displaced quite forward and his back shifted quite posteriorly. This makes his lower back area the spot where the two shifts meet, shear and compress each other.

You may decide that you need to neutralize that pattern, before working on his back. When practitioners work the symptomatic area alone, the client will often feel the change, the release of the knots. After a while, however, the rest of the body's pattern can diminish that good result and recreate the same stressful symptoms.

Perhaps a whole-body assessment could give the information necessary to determine what is the primary and secondary driver in creating the limitation. This could provide a guide for sequencing the treatment, for the most optimal result.

Knowing how to see the whole-body pattern, instead of one isolated symptom or area, may provide the information on what secondary areas may be contributing to the primary area of interest.

Asymmetry in the body is a given, but the compensations to deal with injury, habits, stresses and demands of life can exaggerate these body patterns.

Aston theory and concepts: Part 2

Being in the field of bodywork and movement is rewarding because we educators generally can assist people to neutralize or lessen their challenging patterns. This success often provides new found hope for the students and clients.

Your 'seeing' skills will be useful at any stage of the process: to see where someone starts from and how they change with each session, often becoming more neutral and more vital. You often hear them say, 'I never thought I would feel this much better again.'

As you continue to train your 'seeing' skills, to see the whole-body pattern, you will have more options to help people learn to use their 'best body for now'. This information facilitates problem-solving rather than perhaps old ideas of telling clients how to hold themselves correctly on the Pilates reformer or in yoga.

There is always an available (even if minimal is needed) range of motion that keeps the body in more ease, while allowing the symptoms of the body to be massaged through movement as well.

Her story: At age 2, this client had surgery to remove a tumor on her spine, T5 to T10. The tumor was removed successfully. While she has certain limitations from this history, notice how great a change occurs from before and after one session at our student clinic.

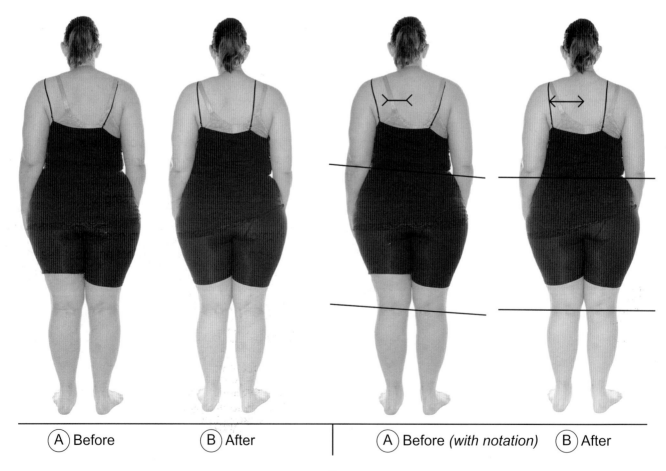

(A) Before   (B) After   (A) Before *(with notation)*   (B) After

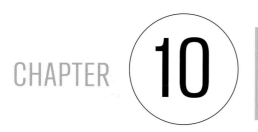
Principle 6: Gravity and ground reaction force (GRF)

The interaction of alignment, dimension, gravity and GRF

To understand the effect of body segments on one another, one must understand the consequential influences of forces. Once you identify the alignment pattern, you can understand which forces affect the skeleton and soft tissues more positively or negatively. Understanding forces will give you more information about your client's pattern and how improving the alignment (therefore neutralizing the negative effect of forces acting on their structure), can decrease their symptoms.

When forces act on the body, they create stress within the body's tissues. In response to these forces, the affected segment often changes in length, depth, width or shape and position (often referred to as *deformation*). Whether the result of the stress is positive or negative is determined by how the body interacts with these forces.

Gravity

Gravity is a continuous force that attracts any body of mass to the center of the Earth. As the Earth's mass is so much greater than that of the human body, we feel the continuous pull of gravity, toward the center of the Earth. It is this gravitational pull that gives the body its sense of weight and often, sense of effort.

1) Experience this: while sitting or standing, raise one arm up as through pointing to the sky; leave the elbow slightly flexed then rotate the hand and forearm, as if screwing in a light bulb. Feel the ease or effort of the motion.

2) Lift your other arm out, so it is parallel to the floor. As you hold it out straight, notice how you feel the increased effort for this arm, as compared to the one that is raised vertically. Now, add the same motion as in #1 (rotating the hand and forearm), to sense the effort needed.

3) Now do the same motions with both arms — one up and the other one out.

Extra effort is required for #2 because there is more surface area in the horizontal arm for gravity to pull on, as opposed to the vertical arm.

This sense of increasing gravitational pull is felt by many people as they age. Sometimes it feels as though the pull of gravity requires a stronger effort to resist. Gravity can also feel much stronger for a person with different tasks and limitations.

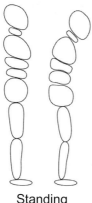
Standing

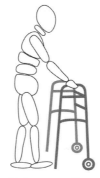
Using a walker

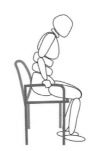
Getting up from a chair

Example

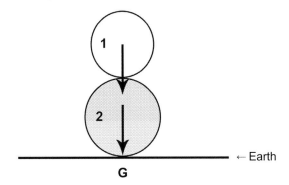

Observe these two ball shapes:

* #1 and #2 are lined up and are being pulled toward the center of the Earth. Since #1 is being pulled down onto #2, #1 adds weight to #2.

* If #1 is heavier than #2, or #2 is very pliable, the effect of #1 would increase the compression on #2 and change its shape; decreased in height, but wider and deeper.

On the previous page, we experienced that the sense of gravity is lesser when holding one arm up vertically in line with the pull of gravity, and feels greater when the arm is held out horizontally, across the field of gravity. This is because the amount of surface area for gravity to pull on is greater with the horizontal arm.

Think about this in terms of this illustration:

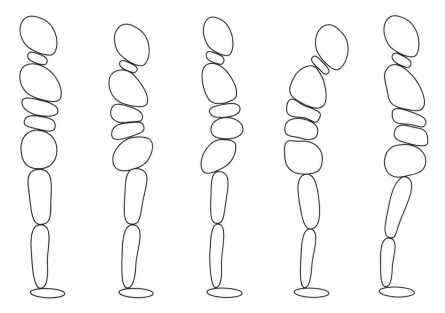

ᵊement of certain body segments increases the pull of gravity on that added surface area. In this sense, a ⁻rience more weight or exert more effort on the lower back, from the chest leaning back or forward.

Ground reaction force (GRF)

How I came to know about ground reaction force (fondly referred to as the 'upside of gravity').
Until the late 1980s, one way I referred to neutralizing the pull of gravity was by the 'push off'. I experienced that, when I pushed off the ground, it made any motion easier. I think anyone who lifts or pulls or pushes off the ground (like dancers, gymnasts, soccer players, weightlifters, etc.) must know about this magic. I had already been teaching this 'push off' concept for 16 years, when I then met Darlene Hertling.

Darlene Hertling, P.T., was taking training sessions with me in Seattle. At the time, she was head of the Physical Therapy department at University of Washington. She came to me after class one day and said, 'You know, that "push off" you love so much does have a name.' It does? 'Yes, it is called Ground Reaction Force.' I was so excited and looked it up immediately.

I find that most people still do not know about this helpful force. You can use it to increase strength, endurance, and balance in relation to gravity. Here are some basic ideas to demonstrate the importance of the interplay between the force of gravity (G) and ground reaction force (GRF).

Newton's third law, the law of action and reaction, states that every force has an opposing counterforce. The opposing force to gravity is known as ground reaction force (GRF). It is the force exerted up from the ground on any object in contact with it. In a sense, this force pushes toward the stars. The magnitude of GRF exerted on us is directly proportional to the amount of weight we apply, as we stand or push on the Earth. It

is the same physics for a large building, pushing down on the Earth, and the Earth pushing back on it.

Our interaction with these opposing forces can determine whether our body segments work effortlessly with one another or with increased effort. When gravity interacts with GRF, as in Newton's law, the two forces are equal in magnitude and opposite in direction. In movement therapy terms, this is often interpreted as resisting gravity, by holding the head and chest up against the pull, which ultimately increases effort and restricts motion.

From my perspective, if we also add the element of varying time to this equation, one can consider these as dynamically alternating forces. Students can be taught how to recycle one force into another. The interplay of gravity and GRF increases the opportunity for the positive use of compression and distraction, where the joints and tissues can be lubricated/hydrated and nutrients exchanged. We can also use GRF to our advantage while performing certain tasks, to help decrease compressive forces in the body and maximize the body's internal volume.

As students or patients are introduced to GRF, they are able to neutralize many of the negative effects of gravity on the body. We can utilize GRF by pushing down onto the surface on which we are supported. If we land on a hard surface, the cement will show little displacement due to the rigidity of the surface. When the upward force is not resisted by a hard surface (like the ground), the net result is a movement upward can that help lengthen the body, or raise the arm up, for example. When we push onto that hard surface, we may find ourselves lifted up or jumping because of no resistance.

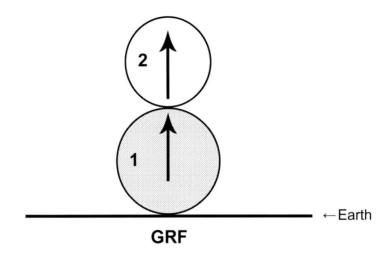

Example: The ground is pushing on ball #1, and ball #1 is pushing up on ball #2.

• If #1 is heavier than #2 or the force of push is greater, #2 will elevate (tensile force).

• If these two balls are pliable, #2 may change shape and have increased length and decreased width.

Let's look at shapes (that will soon become body segments), in relationship to gravity (G) and GRF:

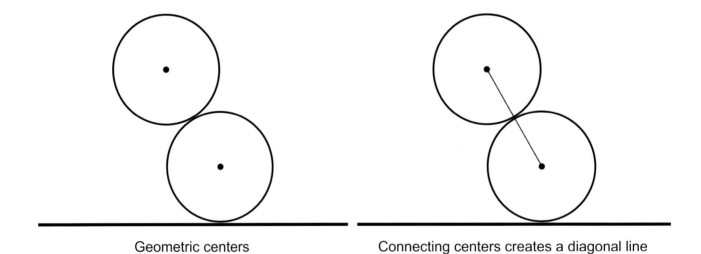

| Geometric centers | Connecting centers creates a diagonal line |

Connecting the dots to lines will demonstrate the angles, and therefore directions, of gravity and GRF.

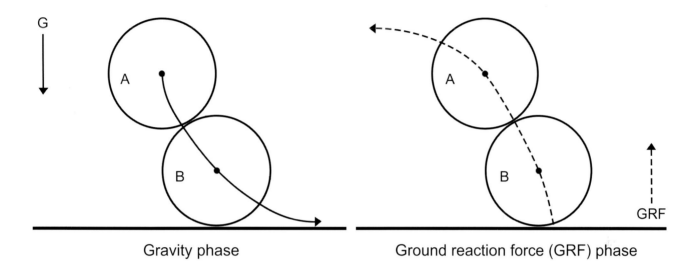

Gravity phase   Ground reaction force (GRF) phase

In this example, **A** will push **B** down and to the right side in G (gravity) phase. In GRF phase, **B** will push **A** up and to the left side.

Conclusion: **A** and **B** are in the same position for both examples, but G and GRF forces are translated in opposite directions.

The combined effect of gravity and GRF

Simply looking at these objects in relation to each other, we see that some are more directly aligned, and others are in a diagonal relationship. In terms of gravity, the more direct alignment naturally translates to easier balance. Before you apply these ideas more specifically to bodies, think about some of the effects that one object will have on another, given different alignments.

Imagine that these shapes (below) are three-dimensional. Look at the shapes with attention to the direction and influence of gravity and GRF. Notice how the placement (shift) of one segment to its adjacent segment determines the angle of the force.

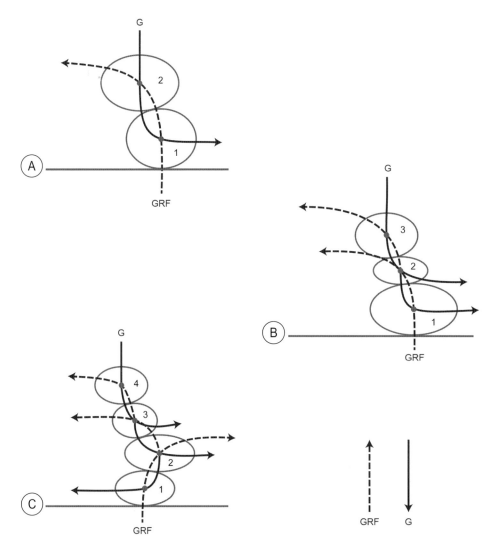

In example **C**, notice the consequence of #2's placement on #1 and to #3, in the opposite direction. This demonstrates how #2 is stressed in both G and GRF phases. If this body segment were the lower back, the person might experience severe pressure there, because the stress from both G and GRF is intensified at that juncture.

Think about any racquet sports you watch or play, or even billiards and golf. In each of these the ball is hit by a piece of equipment. You, plus the added strength and size of the racquet or club, hit the ball with a goal in mind. Ideally, you want to control its direction and speed.

In the case of billiards, those who are very good at it can intentionally aim to hit one ball at such a precise point that it will hit another ball or ricochet, so that it lands specifically where they intend – into a pocket. They use their force, with direction and speed, for a desired result.

But, when it comes to your body, the greater the ricochet effect of translating gravity and GRF in opposite directions, the greater the negative consequences on the body.

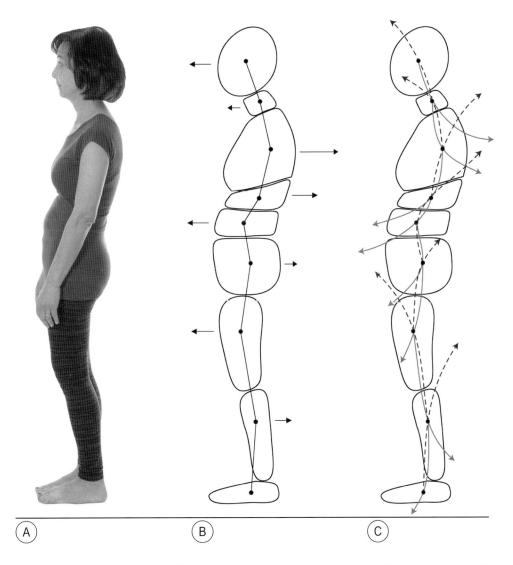

A   B   C

In B, notice how the segmental centers shift forward and back: the arrows visually confirm this pattern. In C, you can see how the G and GRF forces double the effect as they travel through the segments in both directions.

Effects from combined forces and direction

If all the segments of the body were in 'perfect alignment', the force of gravity would run directly down through each center of mass and each segment would directly add weight to the segments below it. This is not often the case. It is important to note that, as a segment is shifted out of alignment, the displaced segments are no longer subject to purely vertical forces, but have additional forces to contend with. These are compression, tensile, shear and torsion (rotational) forces. As these forces are exerted on our neuro-musculoskeletal system, many consequences can arise.

If you imagine the body's segments as spheres, you can see that every segment's misalignment affects the segment below and above it.

Compression forces
If the forces acting on the body's segments are directed toward each other, acting along the same line, they create compression. The compression results in strain, which can shorten and widen the structure.

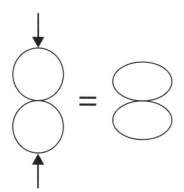

Example: As we age, people often lose height. Some of this has to do with reduced tone, but also compression forces of the segments above, loading segments below.

Tensile forces
If the forces acting on the body are directed away from each other, in opposite directions and along the same line, they create tensile distractive forces, or stretch. Prolonged tensile stress can also result in strain, which can elongate and narrow the segment.

Shear forces

If the forces acting on the body segments are in opposition to each other, the misaligned forces create shear. Shear strain causes a positional change in the segments in line with the path of the force.

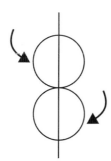

Example: An injured pelvis pushed back and chest pushed forward, creating shear force and changing the shape between the two segments.

Torsion

If the forces acting on the body twist around an axis, they create torque or torsion, commonly known as rotation.

Example: This illustration could be an example of the pelvis being rotated forward, left to right, and the chest rotated forward, right to left.

The structure receives a combination of shear, tensile and compressive forces. The stiffness, elasticity, plasticity and strength of our bones, ligaments, tendons, muscles, joint capsules and connective tissue are tested by all the above forces. The change in any segment's shape (deformation) depends on the amount of force and the type of tissue upon which the forces are applied.

Exercise 10.1

Look at the following photos and silhouettes. Quickly look at one view, say the front or the back.

1) What draws your attention?

2) Do you see:
   a) shearing displacement;
   b) compressions;
   c) rotation (torsion);
   d) change in dimension?

3) What do you see that gives you this information?

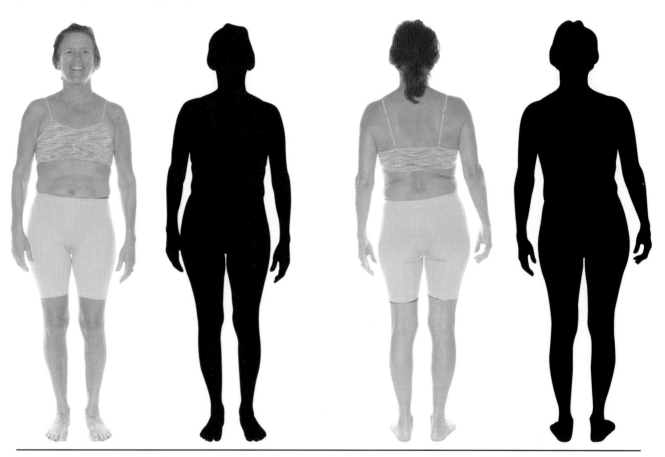

Front   Back

The effect of gravity

The previous exercises have given you a point of reference for considering the body as having segments with different shapes, sizes, and weights. The weight of each body segment impacts the others because of interaction with the forces of gravity and GRF.

Exercise 10.2

1) Mark the **geometric center** of each of these segments.

2) Connect the centers to show the relationship of the segments to each other. This indicates the alignment of parts in relation to one another. Make a few mental notes about the directions of gravity and GRF.

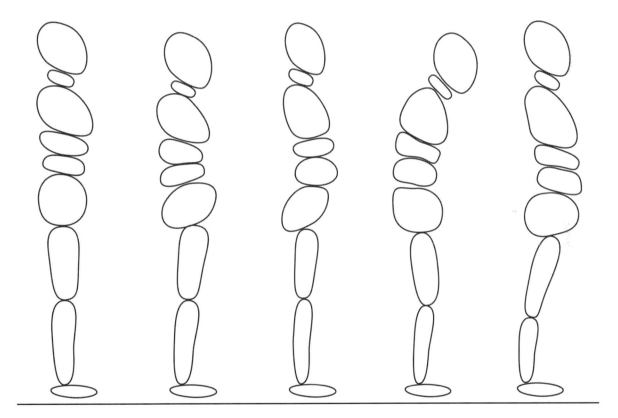

Once you have finished notating, you can see the locations of the stressed areas: segments which receive vector force stresses from both G and GRF phases in opposite directions.

Gravity and GRF – alternating recycling

The Aston principle of dynamic neutral proposes that the body should always be moving, and should not be held still in 'good posture'. This continual movement is aided by using the forces of gravity and GRF, alternating down and up. We teach people to recycle the down into the up and the up into the down. When someone lifts up, against the pull of gravity, they usually fix their position, or go 'on hold'. When someone sustains the lift, to counteract gravity, they are also 'on hold'.

The following landmarks give us reference points for observing the angle of segment relationships in the side view.

Because the body structures are inclined forward (matching the angle of the ribs), there will be a slight downward angle, posterior to anterior.

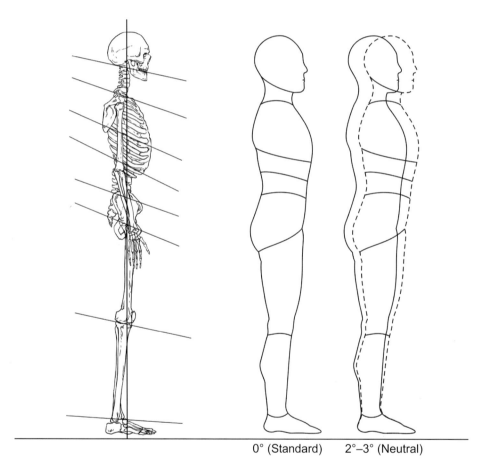

0° (Standard)   2°–3° (Neutral)

For demonstration, the standard plumb line is at 0 degrees, and the dotted line shows the body leaning at 2 degrees, from the front of the ankle. This is the suggested dynamic neutral, moving between 0–5 degrees in stationary balance.

If you were jumping up and down, you'd most likely need to lean by 6–10 degrees.

If you were walking casually, your angle of lean would likely be around 10 degrees.

Exercise 10.3

Without drawing or notating, how do G and GRF move through these two postures?

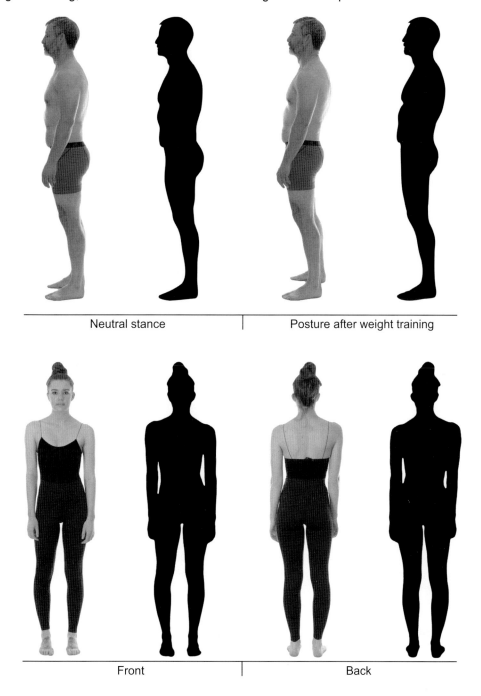

Neutral stance	Posture after weight training

Front	Back

Does any pattern draw your attention here? Which direction might G and GRF take as they move down or up her right leg?

Aston theory and concepts: Part 3

Principle 7: Relationship of alignment and dimension to tone, mobility and holding patterns

Tone

The tone of muscles describes the relative presence or absence of tension, flexibility or resilience within the tissues. This definition of tone must also include the idea of fascia and how the tension or resilience of fascia determine muscle function.

Proportional tone is unique to each individual. It is the amount of tone necessary to stabilize the skeleton and allow for optimal function for each person's range of motion (ROM).

The appropriate tone for any given area (and the whole body) is determined with respect to a person's history of injury, age, activity level, health, and so on. Generally, one would not expect muscle tone to be the same for a 95-year-old and an 18-year-old. There are exceptions, of course. Current research shows impressive tone retention in older people who have kept up their weight training since they were young.

ASTON TONE CONTINUUM											
1	2	3	4	5	6	7	8	9	10	11	12
Hypotonia					Proportional tone					Hypertonia	

Hypotonia is a laxity in the tissues, or less tone than is proportional to the whole body. Hypotonic tissues are slack, overly responsive to forces moving the body, and therefore prone to instability.

Hypertonia is excessive firmness in tissues, or more tone than is proportional to the whole body. Hypertonic tissues are overly contracted or dehydrated, lacking the resilience to respond to the forces of motion, and to expand, stretch, or otherwise change shape, thus overstabilizing the body segment.

When a joint is surrounded by hypotonic tissue, it lacks stability and is at risk of easy displacement. When a joint is surrounded by hypertonic tissue, the joint can become overly stabilized, and normal joint mechanics are altered. The combination of the continuous effort of the hypertonia and instability from the hypotonia can create and reinforce the positions of displacement.

It is challenging to assess the amount of hypertonia and hypotonia in the body, by merely observing it. Adding palpation skills is useful in assessing the tone accurately, to confirm your observations.

Previously, we observed:

1) When body segments are displaced in one direction, they can be balanced or counterbalanced by other segments being displaced in the opposite direction.

2) This balance/counterbalance can create increased dimension in the displaced segment(s), in the same directions as the displacement, thereby decreasing dimension of the segment(s) in the opposite direction.

3) The balance to displacement relationship is influenced by tone. In the photo below, the client is leaning quite forward (anterior) with little displacement posteriorly. How can she do this? Generally, one can achieve balance in this position by increasing tone posteriorly (hypertonicity), as well as sometimes gripping with the toes.

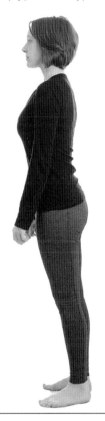

Often, a joint is compressed because its length has been decreased by hypotonicity (not enough tone to stabilize the joint), in the surrounding area. When you add exercise and movement education (to teach the client an improved neutral position that uses the alternating forces of gravity and GRF), the result can be an increase in the length of that segment. This, in turn, can decompress the joint and increase the tone in the surrounding tissues. This result creates a better starting point for deciding and prioritizing what strength exercises or manual therapy techniques would be best to follow.

Beginning strengthening exercises around a joint which is compressed due to displacement and hypertonia may cause additional stress or compression. Too much manual therapy on slackened tissue can increase stress, by making the area even more hypotonic.

Aston theory and concepts: Part 3

Relationship of alignment and dimension to mobility

Mobility is the amount of available motion, or ROM, occurring in a particular joint. It can be observed on a continuum of movement, in relation to the existing condition of the body.

ASTON MOBILITY CONTINUUM

1	2	3	4	5	6	7	8	9	10	11	12

Hypomobility   Proportional mobility   Hypermobility

Proportional mobility is the amount of movement, available at a joint, that is consistent with the joint's normal function, when considering such factors as the individual's age, health and condition.

Hypomobility is limited ROM, a decreased ability to move in response to forces.

Hypermobility is increased ROM, which can produce instability. When a joint is hypermobile, it can be easily displaced and therefore is at risk of injury.

Combinations of tone and mobility

Hypotonia is often accompanied by hypermobility. (The decreased tone encourages too much motion.)

Hypertonia is often accompanied by hypomobility. (The increased tone may restrict motion at the joints.)

People who wish to be strong and toned sometimes undertake extreme workout programs in pursuit of fast results. However, if they work out in a compromised position (e.g., with compressed shoulder or hip joints), this body-use pattern can create strong shear forces in the joints. Over time, this can result in pain, decreased ROM, and wearing down of the skeletal joint surfaces.

When therapists use these ideas, they can evaluate and suggest changes and methods that would be most helpful for the combinations of high or low tone and mobility.

Examples

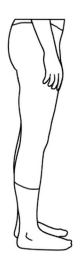

A) A more **neutral position** creates more even tone and mobility through the ankle, knee and hip.

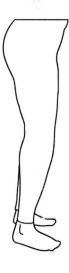

B) The **flexed knee position** increases tone and can decrease mobility through the joints.

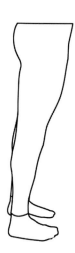

C) The **hyperextended** or **strongly stabilized knee position** can also create uneven tone and mobility through the joints. The displacement of the tibia to femur creates strong anterior to posterior stresses.

Aston theory and concepts: Part 3

Combinations of hypo- and hypertonia and mobility

Let us observe the hypermobility/hypomobility of the hip joint, as it relates to the pull of gravity.

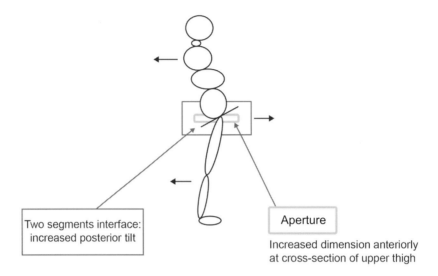

Two segments interface: increased posterior tilt

Aperture

Increased dimension anteriorly at cross-section of upper thigh

The figure shows a forward leg and hip joint with the pelvis tilting back. Notice where these placement directions change: at hip, chest and neck particularly, but also each of the segments. The forward to back shifts create shear forces.

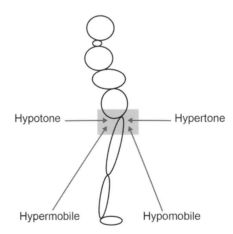

Hypotone — Hypertone

Hypermobile — Hypomobile

Observe how the body placement, the hyper-/hypotonia, and hyper-/hypomobility reinforce the pattern. As one example, the gravitational force would move the upper leg and hip joint forward and push the head of the femur at a sharp angle, into the end of its range. The result of this position would be an overly stabilized hip joint, anteriorly. The gravitational forces would continue to pull the weight of the chest downward, posteriorly. A lack of tone of the posterior pelvic muscles would continue to push the femur forward. This would result in hip joint hypomobility anteriorly and likely hypermobility, posteriorly.

In an older person, this hypermobility could create a risk of subluxation of the hip joint. With gait, a person would need to be particularly cautious if they have had a hip replacement.

Exercise 10.4

Observe this pattern. Imagine the possible combinations of tone and mobility which produced this placement.

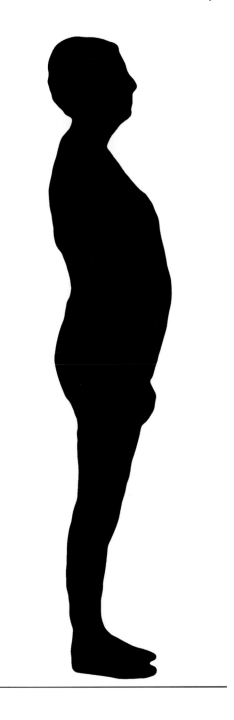

Aston theory and concepts: Part 3

Functional and Structural Holding Patterns continuum

Over the years of working with clients, one of the mysteries that caught my attention was: why did some people achieve major change to their body pattern more quickly than others? Some clients would have major change from just one movement lesson, yet others would need six bodywork sessions to begin to change slightly.

Sometimes, a simple moving meditation exercise would transform the holding pattern for one person and agitate another. What was going on?

I started to evaluate how movement created change in clients' holding patterns. Learning to use their bodies more efficiently was helpful to reduce the amount of stress their previous postures created – but there was more. It seemed as though the movement alone added rehydration, suppleness and increased connection to the surrounding tissues. If I did bodywork on myofascial adhesions in one area, and blended the change through other areas, strong changes were felt and seen throughout the body.

I started to play with the idea that there must be a difference between those holding patterns that were more functional, and those that were more structural. Thus, the continuum – to identify the amount of holding and how anchored it might be.

ASTON HOLDING PATTERN CONTINUUM											
1	2	3	4	5	6	7	8	9	10	11	12
Functional											Structural

The low numbers on the left of this scale represent the more Functional Holding Patterns, progressing in intensity toward the more Structural Holding Patterns.

Functional patterns can arise from such short-term stresses as working to deadlines, bad news, overdoing the yard work or trying to keep up with the son at the gym. They can also simply be someone's posture pattern, which intensifies over time due to the effect of gravity and perhaps lack of tone. These functional patterns might be listed between 1–3. As the numbers approach 4, a client often needs more than one session, one vacation, or a few days of doing what they love to release the pattern of tension. By the mid-range numbers, the client is most likely losing the ability to let go of the pattern.

As the tension pattern becomes more established and in the higher numbers (9–12) there are likely many layers and compensations to the holding pattern. These clients may need a series of therapy sessions, lessons and workouts, to neutralize their restrictions.

A slip on the ice might create a bruise or a broken bone. If the event changed your body's pattern, and if this is then left over time, the functional holding pattern moves up the scale rapidly, toward a structural pattern. Holding patterns that come about from helping your neighbor build his shed over one weekend move up the scale toward structural holding patterns. Habitual patterns of misalignment also tend to become structural holding patterns, over time.

My experiences with these types of holding patterns were intriguing, and made me think more about the continuum from functional to structural holding patterns. Sometimes that continuum starts off functionally – for example, when we decide to 'get into shape'. We start our exercise program, feel the burn, see muscles developing, and do the program every day. And then one day, we experience tremendous pain attempting to lift a 10-pound weight. There are many reasons that could happen (as in we had an injury), but also it can come from not neutralizing the misaligned body pattern after workouts, with each day perhaps taking our body into more compression. The body may be reporting that the compensations we are making, to handle the increase in effort and endurance, have compromised our more neutral alignment pattern.

When someone is able to neutralize functional holding patterns quite quickly, they seem to be fine. As these patterns accumulate, they can become structural holding patterns, embedded in the tissue – and do not always accumulate slowly. A car accident, a serious fall, a trauma, or physical abuse can be instantly transformed by the body into a structural holding pattern. Sometimes, a fleeting event can persist for a lifetime.

I have found bodywork to be one of the fastest ways to neutralize long-term structural holding patterns.

Compensations

Compensations are adjustments the body makes in order to accommodate a lack of balance, space, or specific limitations. Compensations often happen as a subconscious attempt to overcome a limitation. They may increase or decrease segment displacement, or cause one area to overwork while another cannot work or is unable to work hard enough to provide support.

Because the body is mobile, balance is in constant flux. Balance is influenced by habitual ways of moving, repeated actions or activity, and by specific limitations. The inability to bear weight, because of a broken toe or ankle sprain for example, will cause the body to adjust or develop compensations in order to maintain a certain amount of function and balance.

Sometimes the source of an impact trauma creates an emotional response (e.g., loss, fear, anger). This is an example of when the original cause, emotional or physical, is the action that creates a reaction in the body which, in turn, creates the need for compensations.

There are various ways in which the body absorbs the physical and emotional history that may cause misalignments. One option is for the muscles to increase their effort to hold segments in place and balance, with increased tone. Another option is to form adhesions in the myofascial structures, to help support or reinforce segments which are out of alignment. Both of these options lead to uneven tension and tone around the joints that, in turn, lead to uneven patterns of movement, and strain. Often this cannot be seen in photos but can be palpated. We teach therapists to feel myofascial restrictions, increased or decreased tone and joint hypermobility and hypomobility.

As we have seen throughout this book, the familiar scenario of displacement of one segment can require the counterbalance of another segment, in an opposing direction.

For example, when you see a lateral shift of the pelvis to the direction of the right side, you might see a lateral shift of the shoulders/upper chest in the opposite (left) direction. This counterbalance often occurs in order to maintain overall balance of the body's segments around its center.

We have talked about counterbalance by displacing segments in the opposite direction from one another. Another way to counterbalance a segmental displacement is to increase the tension or tone of another segment. For example, I may shift my pelvis forward but, rather than shift my chest back to counterbalance, I may increase my abdominal muscle tone to hold me in a more direct alignment or 'good posture'.

A long-term goal for teachers and therapists might be to facilitate our clients to restore more central balance of their body segments. For example, to offer bodywork and movement sessions to lessen some of the holding patterns/restrictions that cause the body to be unnecessarily asymmetrical or in discomfort. The treatment plan might allow the right and left sides to be more proportionate, without needing to add unnecessary effort to hold the improvements.

Symmetry is often linked with the term balance. This can imply an arrangement of segments to be equal on either side of a median line, to be a mirror image of each other. Balance can also mean the way in which dissimilar or opposing forces offset each other.

I define **balance** as 'the moment to moment negotiation of asymmetrical differences'.

It seems obvious that most bodies are in balance, meaning that our body compensations keep us standing. However, this may not produce the best available alignment for the short or long term. Life experiences certainly have a way of imparting specific consequences that take us somewhat off track, from whatever we think is ideal. Generally, I think there is always a way to find improvement.

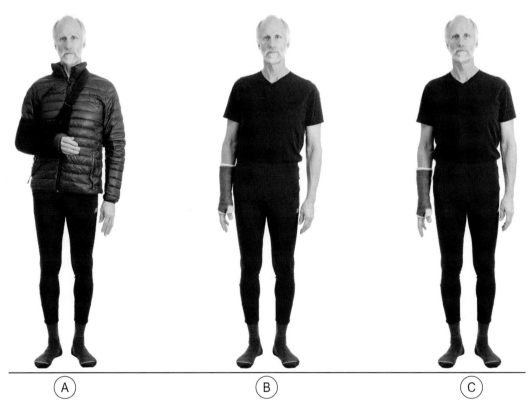

Examples

A) The client is pictured after a fall from a 10-foot ladder. The cast went above the elbow to hold the arm in flexion.

B) This is the second cast. You can see a tendency has set in, from being in the first cast, to shift his chest to the left, to counterbalance the cast.

C) Several weeks later, you can see how he has neutralized his pattern from the fall.

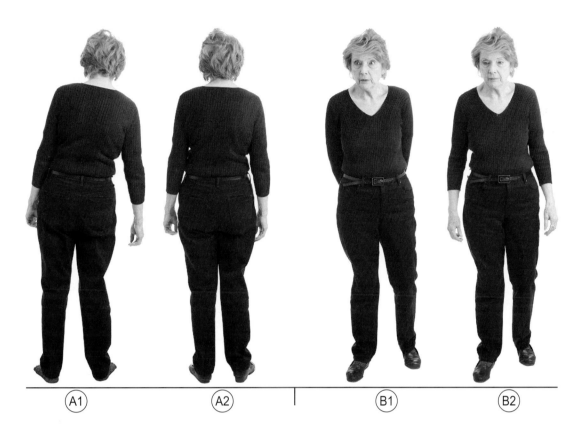

(A1)   (A2)   (B1)   (B2)

As a child of nine, this client had an illness that left her with severe limitations, particularly in her right leg. The result is a shortened right leg length. As she started and progressed through her sessions, she had fewer compensations and a new ability, with knowledge of how to use her best available body in gait. The releases in her body allow her a new range of motion.

A1 and B1: With her leg length, notice that when she steps right, she displaces her upper trunk to the right, to negotiate.

A2 and B2: Here, an insert in her shoe compensates for her leg length discrepancy, allowing her to step with more even height on her right leg and resulting in less displacement of her trunk. Instead of each step borrowing from her energy (because of the need for effort), this gait pattern provides her with energy and strength, while walking.

Positive effects of balanced posture

1) The placement of body segments allows for optimal ROM at the joints.

2) When the body's weight-bearing is more direct, the body can positively utilize the compression and distraction forces of gravity and GRF.

3) The effort for work (muscle use) is more evenly distributed throughout the body.

4) Because the three dimensions are more optimal, the internal volume of a segment is more optimal, which improves the functions of breath, digestion, circulation, etc.

5) The muscle tone is strong enough to support the body segments and stabilize the structure, and also, resilient enough to allow full ROM.

As your observation skills become more precise, you can recognize when each client finds their unique balanced posture. This balance will be dynamic, in continuous motion, and will change from moment to moment.

As the body approaches its optimal posture, the position, space, effort, movement and physiology are more optimal. The consequences of these relationships will determine the body's ability to feel increased awareness, support, stability, resiliency, and mobility, as well as have the possibility of a full range of expression of thoughts and emotions.

Sometimes body patterns create shapes that may or may not be accurate reflections of expression. For example, someone experiencing grief may take on a slouched posture. Perhaps they took on the pattern many years ago and it has remained with them. Sometimes, people will interpret someone's patterns and relate to them accordingly. People are unique in their complexity. Even if people have had similar experiences, the how, the when, and the content of those experiences combine to make the results quite different and unique to each person.

It is always rewarding to facilitate a student or client to lessen their holding of an old pattern, and enable them to have more freedom to express themselves.

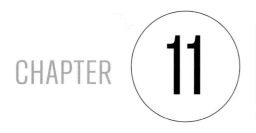
Physical benefits

People seek bodywork treatment to neutralize the negative effects of trauma, injuries, surgeries, and accumulated stress from body use and habitual expression patterns. They understand that the accumulated effects of these dictate their current amount of ease, strength, and flexibility, and consequently their long-term quality of life. Many therapists appreciate how Aston Seeing Skills help them to teach clients about their body patterns. Therapists then can educate, and not just fix isolated problems.

Therapists say that Aston Seeing Skills:

1) Facilitate diagnosis by prioritizing and/or sequencing treatment.

2) Provide a system for refining skills in recognizing compromised relationships of one body part to another.

3) Offer information about areas of the body that are overutilized or underutilized, while performing an activity.

4) Help in applying and integrating these concepts with other learned techniques.

5) Assist the physical therapist in treatment and in teaching efficient patterns of functional movement, which helps prevent the recurrence of pain.

6) Assist in designing a treatment plan that establishes adequate support in the body for a specific task, such as an appropriate base of support in standing to facilitate reaching.

7) Are applicable to everyone from the elite athlete to the neurologically or physically challenged patient.

8) Expand the occupational therapist's ability to analyze and identify the client's body pattern and how it contributes to their symptom(s), for more effective intervention.

9) Support efficient use of therapy time to educate patients in optimal use of their bodies, while respecting existing limitations.

10) Empower therapists to view the body holistically, each part exhibiting a cause-and-effect relationship. This helps them to identify and treat deficits that interfere with the activities of daily living.

11) Allow them to identify which areas of the musculoskeletal system are compressed, overextended, decreased in dimension, hypermobile or hypomobile.

12) Help them demonstrate how a body pattern contributes to fatigue, overuse syndromes, and pain.

13) Provide for better understanding and communication of the relationships between soft tissue restrictions and body alignment.

14) Help the personal trainer see where the client needs to increase or decrease tone to improve alignment, stabilize good posture, increase strength and improve function.

15) Help in the design of exercises that are based on an individual's unique structural pattern, decreasing the risk of injury.

16) Increase the ability to see body patterns and help clients achieve optimal improvement, by observing the individual pattern before the exercise (pre-test) and how the exercise subsequently changed that pattern.

Psychological benefits

In addition, psychotherapists have found that understanding some elements of the relationship of physical or postural expression to a person's internal reality or psyche can offer tools for assisting a client's progress. Alignment and dimension combine to give the body its shape, which can reflect or store elements of history, personality and style of communicating. Psychotherapists often see clients when they are stuck in a loop of experience or behavior that reinforces itself with a corresponding body pattern. The capacity to perceive, and perhaps enable the client to perceive, self-expression in terms of alignment and dimension can be useful in:

1) Providing tangible guidelines to see and work with the whole person.

2) Identifying and integrating the expression of particular emotional states or self-images in the body (e.g., to differentiate an internal pattern, such as fear, grief, from an external expression, such as anger).

3) Seeing how a body pattern may be expressing a historical moment that has or has not been worked through.

4) Recognizing how a familiar body pattern may restrict certain new expressions or experiences.

5) Helping the therapist know when to refer a patient for work on physical patterns, in order to facilitate the psychotherapeutic process.

Additional information for observing posture

You can gain even more insight by asking your client to stand in different ways. Ask your client to:

1) Stand in their best posture. This demonstrates learned postural positions.

2) Stand in their casual stance. This demonstrates compensation tendencies.

3) Stand as usual with weight on both feet. This can demonstrate the tendency of the body to be more centered over the left or right foot, or over the heels or balls of the feet.

4) Stand on both feet with the eyes closed. This demonstrates the change in balance when the client is not using the eyes to secure postural position.

Using photos and videos

Visual references are useful for therapists and clients.

1) Benefits to therapists:

   a) Recording posture in all four views at the beginning of treatment, as a reference point.

   b) Comparing changes throughout the client's sessions.

   c) Documenting results at the end of treatment.

   d) Determining the next step in treatment and observing certain tendencies in results that may indicate an area that may have been overlooked.

2) Benefits to clients:

   a) Encouraging participation in the session.

   b) Educating. Some people have never seen themselves from the side view or back view. This is often an eye-opening experience. Some clients prefer not to see their photos. In this case, it is better to keep the photos in your file until significant visual changes occur. Then you can have the client observe the difference, if they wish.
   If the client has low self-esteem or is highly self-critical, perhaps you could use tracing paper to make a ball body drawing to show them instead of their photos, in case they only see their body negatively.

Different ways to use photos

A) Overlay with tracing paper to outline the segments and observe alignment and dimension. This creates an abstract body drawing.

B) Use dental floss as the plumb line to easily identify displacements.

C) Overlay with tracing paper to notate placement and dimension or to notate placement and dimension on a body chart. Transfer the notations onto a body chart.

D) Turn the photo upside down for a different perspective of how the client would be able to balance if standing on their head and ask would they fall forward or backward?

E) Observe one isolated segment (e.g., the head or foot) by covering the rest of the body with a piece of paper. As you slide the paper along (one segment at a time), imagine or draw what you think the position of the other body segments would be, in neutral. Compare your drawing with the photo.

F) Instead of drawing lines to connect segmental centers on a chart or a transparency, draw the lines directly on the photo. Later, you can transfer the lines to a body chart.

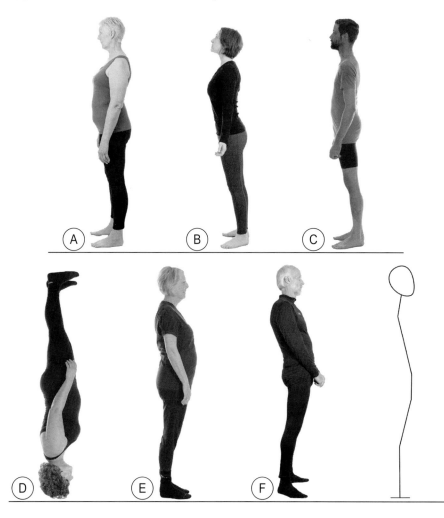

186

Session sequence flowchart

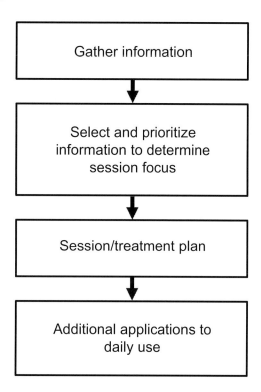

Gather information

Select and prioritize information to determine session focus

Session/treatment plan

Additional applications to daily use

Observation sequence

The following is a suggested sequence to help you prioritize and summarize the information you gather.

1) What view gives you the most information?

2) What area catches your attention first (Area 1)?

3) What is the relationship of Area 1 to another body area (Area 2)?

4) What is their relationship to the whole body?

5) What are the consequences of the above on dimension?

6) What are the possible consequences of tone and mobility on the body, in relation to the alignment or dimension?

7) What are the possible challenges for the client with this pattern?

8) How does this information relate to the client's focus, history, symptoms, lessons and exercises?

Integrating seeing into your practice

Sample session sequence and form

This session sequence may be useful in designing your sessions, lessons and exercises.

1) Gather information
    a) Client's focus: interest, motivation.
    b) History: past injuries, surgeries, structural limitations, current symptoms and body usage (e.g., athlete, mother, job).
    c) Pre-test: stance, gait, ADL, bending, lifting.
        Options for the therapist to take:
            Photo – four views
            Video – two views
            Video action – standing, bending, tennis serve, golf swing, gait, etc.
        For the client:
            Initial self-awareness of posture or function for post-session comparison.
    d) Palpation and body mapping (we train therapists to add these additional skill sets).
    e) Notation on body chart: to confirm observations and assure the whole-body pattern is accurately assessed and notated, and to be able to demonstrate the visual record to the client.

2) Select and prioritize information to determine the session focus and plan

3) Session/treatment plan
    a) Objective
    b) Content:
        Modalities
        Bodywork
        Exercise
        ADLs
    c) Result: post-test (compare with pre-test)

4) Additional applications to daily use: ADLs, sports, etc.

5) Summary (for the client; anchor with a specific and simple cue to retain change).

One Sample Session Form

Client's name _____ Date: _____

Subjective (Client's focus):
Circle area(s) of complaint

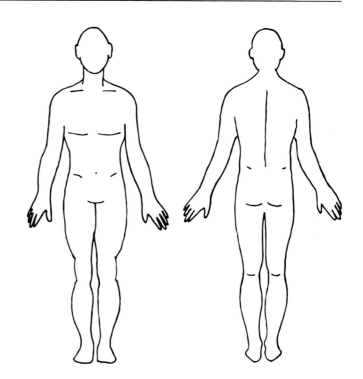

Objective (Your observation of
alignment, dimension, etc.)**:**

Assessment (Hypothesis)**:**

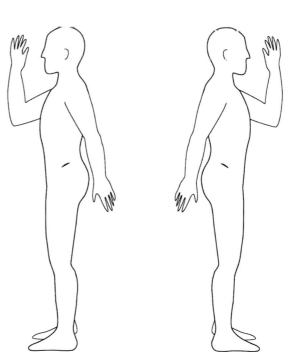

Plan (Session sequence):

Integrating seeing into your practice

Learning review

Exercise 11.1

Observe this body drawing and answer the following questions.

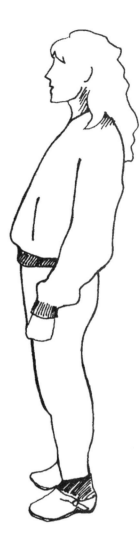

1) What draws your attention first?
   a) The alignment
   b) The dimension
   c) The expression

2) What segment draws your attention the most?

3) That segment (from question 2, above) is in relationship to which other segment(s)?

4) What primary track does this body pattern create?
   a) Pattern of displacement – anterior to posterior, right to left and up to down
   b) Dimensional changes
   c) Extension/flexion pattern
   d) Rotational pattern

5) When you have identified your primary track, what do you think might be the major consequences?
   a) The biomechanical forces of:
      • Compression
      • Tensile
      • Shear
      • Torsion
   b) The path of direct/indirect weight-bearing
   c) The translation of the forces of gravity and GRF
   d) The increase and decrease of hypertonia and hypotonia
   e) Possible challenges this person may experience

Once you answer the questions above, you can draw initial conclusions. Checking the client's complaint, reported at the beginning of the session, will help you progress.

Sample assessment

1) The alignment (placement) draws my attention.

2) The posterior alignment of the upper chest is the segment that draws my attention the most.

3) The posterior alignment of the upper chest is in relationship to the anterior pelvic placement.

4) The body pattern creates an increase in the length of the anterior chest, in relationship to a decreased length of the low back.

5) Possible challenges:

   a) Compression or impact to the lower back
   b) Decreased breathing capacity in the posterior chest
   c) Decreased support for weight of the head and therefore, increased tension on posterior neck, upper back and shoulders
   d) Shear through the viscera and the diaphragm

6) Compare your assessment to the client's complaint or focus. She might have included one of these statements:

   a) Low back pain at work.
   b) I always feel tense and tight, mainly in my neck.
   c) I am losing overall body height.

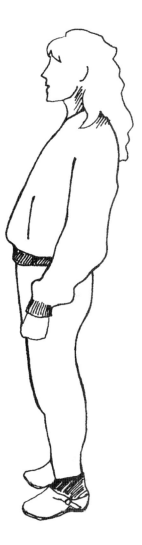

In relation to this illustration, there are two patterns that sometimes are overlooked.

1) The combined anterior placement of the hip and the pelvis (PSIS) tilting back moves the ischial tuberosities close to the femur, which decreases the posterior depth of the hip joint, and therefore decreases support for the posterior depth of the segments above, particularly the back.

2) Sometimes, therapists assess a client as having an increased lumbar lordosis when actually it appears more lordotic because of the extreme posterior placement of the lower and upper chest, combined with anterior placement of the hip joint.

Exercise 11.2

Start by assessing the outlined and segmented body drawing first, then compare to the information you glean from looking at the illustration.

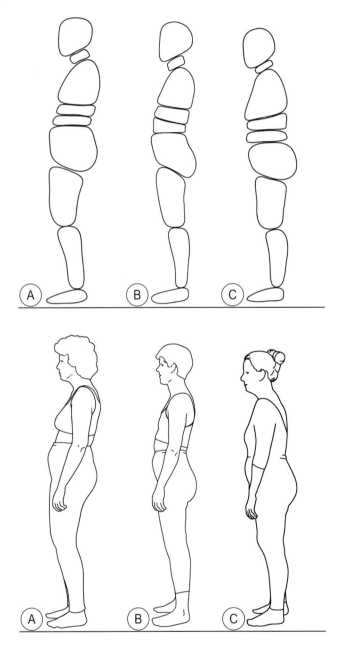

By now, perhaps you are able to assess as much information from a photo as the outline drawing. If you find it's easier to see segmental relationships with the outlined body, continue outlining the body first, from your photos onto tracing paper. Either way, it's a helpful practice to discover and confirm your assessment.

Exercise 11.3

Part 1: For the three people below, observe the whole-body pattern and consider possible consequences of the segmental relationships.

1) Which view gives you the most information, front or side?

2) In that view, what segment gives you the most information?

3) What is the relationship between that segment and another segment or segments?

4) What might be the consequences (stress, pain, decreased ROM, strength, etc.)?

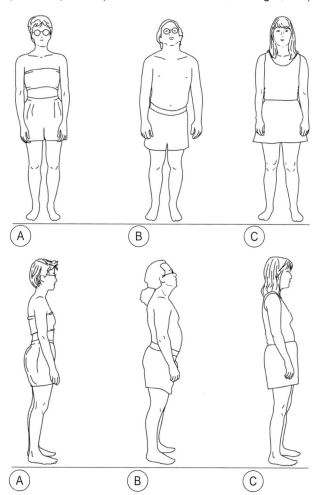

Part 2: For these three people, select your initial track:

1) Placement: right–left

2) Placement: anterior–posterior

3) Flexion–extension

A body can appear to be in good posture (with its key landmarks in line); however, if a person has decreased dimension in the anterior chest (compression, lost depth) in relation to increased depth and length in the posterior chest/back, they could experience increased compression and shear forces in the low back.

Communicating with your client

How you communicate with your clients will determine not only what they learn, but also how they feel about themselves when they hear the information or receive the treatment.

Communication guidelines

1) Use descriptive words rather than interpretive words (e.g. 'Your back is shorter than your front, which can create stress in your low back,' rather than 'Your back is compressed' or 'Your chest slouches').

   a) This enables you to communicate with less emotionally charged words, making the problem more manageable.

   b) This enables clients to be more involved in problem-solving, with less judgment.

2) Designing the pre-test

   a) Include the client in the process of discovering elements that contribute to their discomfort or area of interest, engaging their participation, curiosity and questioning.

   b) Depending on the client's self-awareness, have them pre-test and post-test on a few examples:

   - Count the seconds it takes and the amount of breath they can take in a deep inhalation.

   - Where do they feel the greatest area of weight-bearing on the feet, in standing or on impact in gait?

   - Check the range of motion of any specific joint in reaching, side bending, etc.

3) When coaching or teaching, watch your own placement/posture in relation to the client.

   a) Some people feel uncomfortable when being talked to as you face them.

   b) Standing beside the client can feel more collaborative, so you are both looking at the assessment together.

   c) Demonstrating the pattern in question, yourself, allows clients to see the math and posture and consequence of stress, without the judgment associated with only being observed.

At this time, take a moment to observe the client below. Use the observation sequence here to guide you.

Observation sequence

1)   What view gives you the most information – the front, back or sides?

2)   What area draws your attention first?

3)   This area (from question 2) is in relationship to what other area?

4)   What relationship does this area have with the rest of the body?

5)   What is the consequence on dimension?

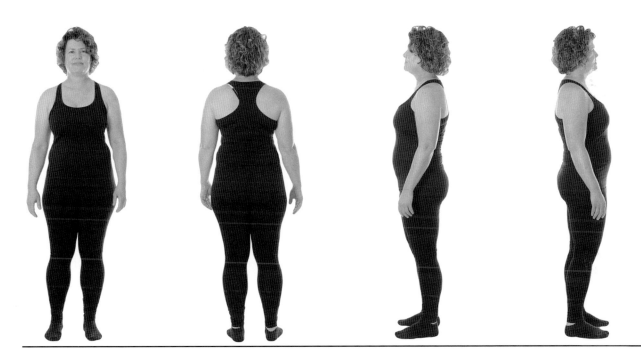

Exercise 11.4: Test your seeing skills

1) Looking at the following figures, can you now identify why the top segments (upper trunk, neck, and head) do not belong to these lower body patterns?

2) Before you look at the next page, see if you can give two reasons why they do not match.

3) Now, look at the next page and compare these figures with their correct body patterns.

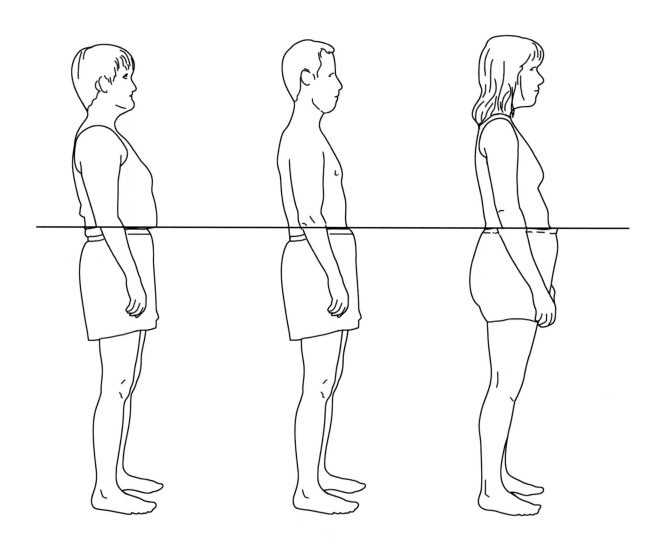

These are the mismatched lower body patterns from the previous page:

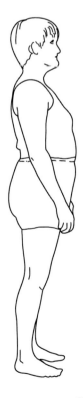
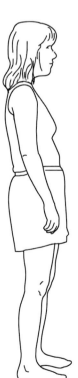
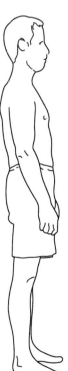

These are the real patterns. Can you see how the upper and lower bodies match?

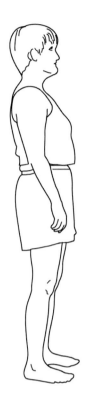
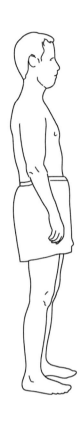
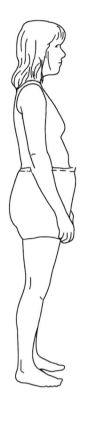

Putting it all together

Making the connection between client patterns, their complaints and your notations and assessment

Example 1: Finding the connection between pattern and pain or limitation the client has expressed.

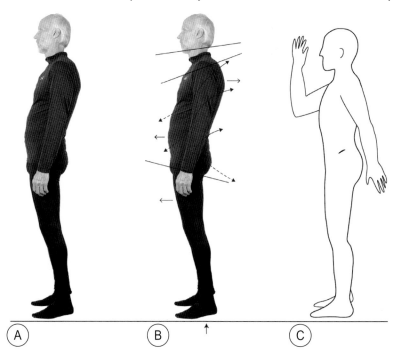

A   B   C

A: Photo of client.
When you look at photo **A**, what draws your attention? Identify the track; is it placement, tilts, rotation or dimension? How does the area you picked relate to another area within the same track?

B: Notate your assessment on **B**.
Can you see where the stresses are increased by his possible pattern? Draw the directions of gravity and ground reaction forces, going from his foot to head and his head to foot. Can you see how the pelvis being forward and the chest being back send the ground reaction force into his low back? And how gravity, from his chest leaning back, pushes his lower chest and abdomen further forward? The consequence of this pattern could create or add to an existing 'low back problem'.

C: Generic body chart.
The body chart is included on the client intake form, along with their history and areas of focus or complaint. You will often have the client complete this form ahead of time, and perhaps email it to you before the session. The complaint usually makes the most sense when you have the photo, the history and your assessment.

This assessment technique can help you and the client make connections between their history, injuries and stressful body usage patterns. This assessment can help the client, and you, to work out solutions for their pain, stress or limitation.

Example 2: Ask your clients how they use their bodies during the day.

You need to see the client's interpretation of how they use their body during the day. They may say, 'Oh, I just sit in a chair all day, at the computer. It is a pretty comfortable chair, but I just sit', but you cannot know what that means without seeing the true interpretation of the task of sitting. How high is the chair, are their knees higher than their pelvis, is the major part of their day spent rotating to the right, to use the printer on the right?

This is sometimes an instant revelation for the practitioner, when the client shows them their setup either in person or with a photo or video of them at work.

People can be uninformed about how things such as chairs, work stations and shoes can dictate their body use, and therefore their posture.

Look at this series of photos. This client said she previously worked as a server in a restaurant and bar. I did think to ask if she had to carry a tray, and that became a big part of her problem at work.

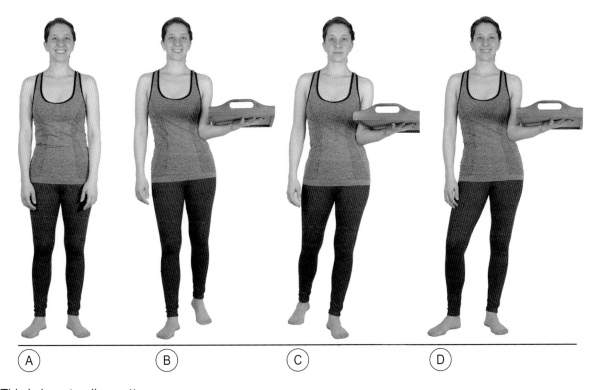

A   B   C   D

A) This is her standing pattern.

B) Carrying a lighter tray.

C) Carrying a heavier tray.

D) Pausing to talk with customers at a table.

Compared to photo **A** without the tray, can you see the effect of her carrying the tray? Her chest is shifted to the right and her pelvis is high on the left.

Example 3: Holding 'good posture'.

We posed this client to demonstrate a certain pattern. His whole-body alignment looks fairly direct, with slight shifts back in his chest and forward in his head.

If you evaluate what draws your attention the most, I believe the loss of dimension in his chest seems obvious. The angle of his pelvis, in posterior tilt, also contributes to diminished support for his chest volume.

Sometimes the client's intake and history form will reveal conditions that might contribute to the chest pattern: asthma, broken anterior ribs that were never set in place, neck surgery that fused his neck in flexion (C2–C4).

This could be a case where the chest has no problem occupying its full volume and depth dimension, but the neck fusion prohibits the posterior neck from lengthening. So, the chin is pushed up, shortening the back of the neck, which pushes the anterior chest down.

These examples could be structural holding patterns or given limitations that need to be worked with. I find that, even with strong structural holding patterns, the practitioner and client can find ways to facilitate more cooperation from the rest of the body segments. Often, the work can change the vectors of impact to be more evenly distributed through the body, instead of stressing the same limited, isolated areas.

While you might be most focused on the dimension of his anterior chest, it turns out that the greatest tension (holding pattern) is in his arms (particularly, his upper arms), resulting from doing landscaping work for years. This arm work may help his chest release more than working on his chest.

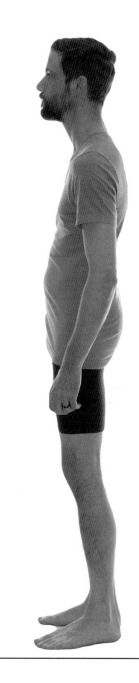

Example 4: Past injuries.

This client looks in more direct alignment, up until the neck and head pattern he is demonstrating for this photo. One could suspect a possible whiplash or injury that might have pushed his neck forward and thrust his head back.

Notating tilts gives visual feedback that his upper ribs are down in front and his scapula is high in the back. The neck is long in front (chin up), and short in the back.

His intake form might state that he had a broken clavicle. This injury may have compressed the front of the chest, and so produced this pattern while he was healing. He may only have become aware of the consequences of this pattern until sometime later, when he started to get spasms in his upper back.

Healing a broken bone not only requires the body to mend the fracture – the process involves all the soft tissues surrounding it too (and often, throughout the whole body). The negative effects of trauma need to be neutralized by working with the soft tissues to reclaim their resiliency and therefore, be able to occupy a more neutral position.

I add this thought because so many people believe that as soon as bones are healed, they are 'good to go'. What happens after that is all too common – the consequences from the original injury may affect many other areas that cannot negotiate the restrictions that remain unless the whole body pattern is addressed.

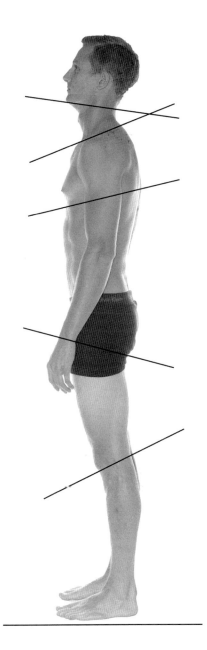

Example 5: Before and after.

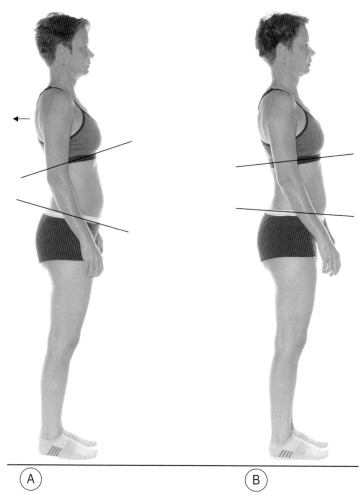

A ⃝   B ⃝

A (before session): In assessing this client's pattern, observing tilts gives us good information. You can see she has an anterior tilt at the iliac crest, a posterior tilt at her xyphoid to T10–11, and that her chest is placed posterior to her midline.

B (after session): After one session in our student clinic, this client was able to neutralize the angle of her pelvis, lessening the posterior lean of her upper chest, to be in more direct alignment over her feet.

As her alignment became more direct in its placement, she gained more dimension – vertical length in her body. She was pleased to feel taller, so of course we had to measure that – and she was. To help support her change, we reminded her to adjust the position of the rear-view mirror in her car – to accommodate her new height.

As segments are able to release the tension that holds them off-center, the body can reclaim more of its natural length, depth and width.

I add this example of gaining length because while practitioners may want to see rotations, shifts and tilts *all* corrected during a session (which may happen), often a session may be more about reclaiming dimension.

Example 6: Extreme patterns.

This illustration is taken from a snapshot that my friend took of her daughter, while they were shopping in a store.

The position of her hyperextended left knee is at such a sharp angle that the weight-bearing from the rest of her body pushes her left knee further back, with each step.

For the moment, start by identifying the placement of segments from her left side. This is obviously not a direct left-side view, as she is rotating to her right. If she were rotating to her left, her left knee would shift even further back.

She is still young enough to lessen this pattern, perhaps even to neutralize most of it, with bodywork, movement education and toning to stabilize a more direct weight-bearing pattern.

It has been my privilege to see so many transformations happen through the decades. It is such an honor to facilitate people to find a better, easier, freer body, that can change their lives and provide them with hope.

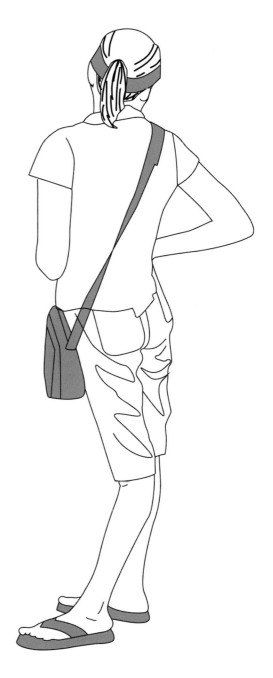

Post-test A

It's time to review your progress! Now that you have completed this book, take a moment to look at the following photo and write down what you see (this is the photo you assessed for the Pre-test, in Chapter 1).

After recording your observations, compare your notes here to those you took at the beginning of the book. Are you seeing differently now?

Answer these questions.

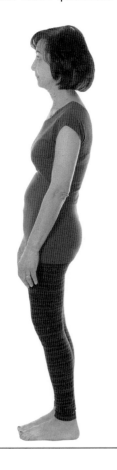

1) What do you see?

2) What do you think this person's complaints might be?

3) What areas might you address in a session or lesson and why?

Notes:

_____

_____

_____

_____

_____

_____

Post-test B

1) Reassess the photos of yourself, from Pre-test B in Chapter 1. Jot down your observations or use tracing paper to record your assessment.

2) Compare this post-test assessment with your pre-test assessment.
   a) How do your pre-test observations compare with your post-test observations?
   b) Does this post-test information change your treatment or lesson plan, from the pre-test?

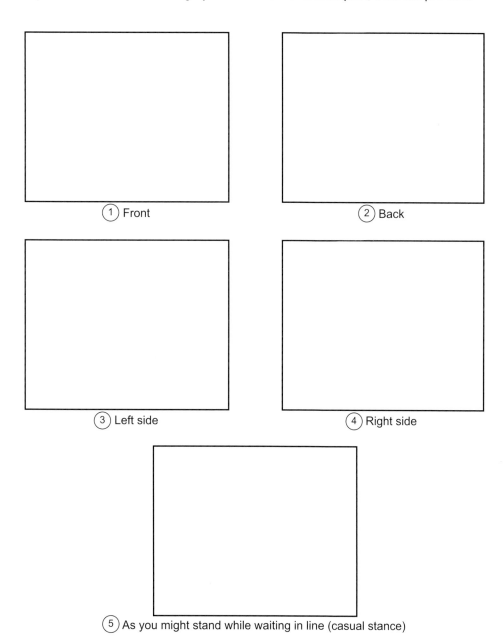

① Front   ② Back

③ Left side   ④ Right side

⑤ As you might stand while waiting in line (casual stance)

Before and after (and 22 years later)

Compare this client's before- and after-session photos from 1996 and 2018.

The left side:

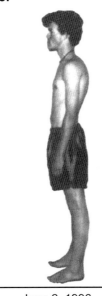 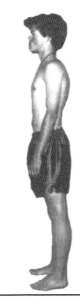 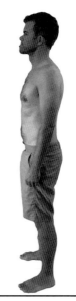

| June 2, 1996 | June 2, 1996 | September 2018 |
| (before his first session) | (after his first session) | (after one session 22 years later) |

The right side:

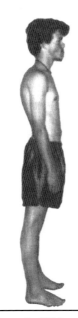 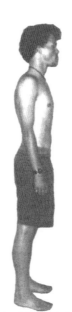 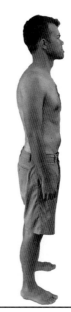

| June 2, 1996 | June 2, 1996 | September 2018 |
| (before his first session) | (after his first session) | (after one session 22 years later) |

Aston Body Mapping

This book provides an introduction to our body mapping. I hope you will practice these tools, to be able to quickly assess and notate the body patterns of your students or clients.

I created and started training therapists in Aston Body Mapping in 1979. In our sessions we include additional notations of hyper- and hypotonicity, and hyper- and hypomobility, by pattern and layer. An example of that process includes: visual assessment, then palpation, along with the client's history, focus and areas of body pain or stress, all notated on their intake form and body map.

Once the observation is combined with palpation, the client's history and interests, the body map will reveal what work is needed where, and the tools to determine the best treatment sequence.

I look forward to progressing and expanding our body mapping theories at another time.

In closing

Just as each client has their own unique physical and emotional history, each postural assessment will be different. Learning how to see helps the therapist pay attention to what the body is saying, in a multitude of different ways. As your seeing skills become more refined, your abilities to discern and guide a client on the path of healing become more effective.

These assessment guidelines provide the information and vocabulary for an ongoing therapeutic conversation. As the client brings new postural awareness into everyday activities, their observations and experiences can offer valuable information for ongoing sessions. Returning to the postural assessment tools in this book is a good way to highlight important insights, reflect on progress, and identify the next steps forward.

When the client experiences how a slight postural adjustment impacts comfort, stress and attitude, a connection opens between mind and body. Posture is no longer a frustrating, static given, it's a fluid, dynamic variable. These transformative 'Aha!' moments empower both practitioner and client, teacher and student: when a client discovers that, rather being held hostage by their posture, they have a choice.

It's easy to see that such moments might be linked to new perspectives on old issues. Just shifting from a braced posture to one that's more resilient, supported and balanced, changes the whole picture for the practitioner as well as the patient.

Integrating seeing skills into your therapeutic practice will deepen your understanding and expand your therapeutic skill. As with any practice, the more you use these assessment tools, the more your own vision and understanding will embrace the body as an expression of one's entire history.

This is quite a significant reality; that the body carries that person's whole life history of accidents, injuries, health, emotion, daily usage and exercise, etc. As therapists, teachers, coaches, we must always be mindful to do our best to see how a suggestion will affect or be tolerated by the whole body.

With good intention, teachers, coaches and therapists sometimes impose an alignment pattern on a body that is 'more correct' or perhaps more 'bilaterally symmetrical.'

As an example: when the running coach can see that the pattern of both feet internally rotating is actually occurring all the way up both legs, to internally rotated hip joints, she would not make an isolated correction of holding the feet in a straight-ahead stride.

When a coach has this skill of seeing, he can appreciate that giving an isolated correction or cue, for the runner to hold her feet straight, might lead to a strain pattern at the foot and ankle and possibly an injury. Isolated areas of focus need to be balanced and negotiated throughout the body.

What might be possible options for your seeing skills of the above pattern? Depending on what patterns you find of tension or lack of tone, you might select from the following examples:

1) A stretching sequence for the adductors is needed, to lessen the internal rotation of the legs.

2) Massage would be helpful, to lessen the tension patterns that pull the legs in.

3) Toning the lateral and posterior muscle groups of the legs, to increase their support for more neutral position and balance of tone.

Let's look at the person's pattern on page 204 again (Post-test A) and see how we might progress our findings, to determine our session focus and sequence.

1) What gets **my attention**:

   • I could focus on the dimension track and the diminished depth of her upper anterior chest.

   • Or, I could focus on the alignment track of the upper leg placed forward of the lower leg, pelvis back, chest further back and head forward.

   • Or, I could focus on the alignment tilts of her pelvis down in back, hip joint slightly high in front and chest down in front and high in back.

2) **Her attention** or complaint might be neck and shoulder stress, which she thinks is the result of her office job and sitting at the desk all day.

3) I now need to explore options for determining what area is more controlling (primary pattern A for this day) and what area seems to be more able to negotiate the primary pattern (secondary pattern B).

4) If you are trained in palpation skills, you can often quickly determine what areas are more controlling, through tension or limitation (perhaps the injury or surgery has altered the available or natural range of motion for a specific area).

5) If you do not have palpation skills, then explore what body areas are more on hold and unable to have a full range of motion.

   • Using the woman on page 204 as the example, ask yourself: Is her pelvis in its posterior tilt, pulling her chest down in front or is her chest pushing down on her pelvis and encouraging it to be in a posterior tilt?

   • You could ask her if she can easily extend and stretch her chest up or is it held down through tension. If it does lift, does this change her pelvis position?

   • You could ask her if she can easily and slightly lift and tilt her pelvis more up and forward. If she has this range, does it also lift her chest up?

6) For the sake of problem solving, let's say she had more range to move her pelvis than her chest. This finding, combined with her focus of her neck and shoulder stress, would lead me to focus on the upper body first, through movement or bodywork.

7) The idea here is to focus on the more controlling area (A), before the area that has more range of motion (B). Currently, the lower area seems to be able to negotiate or accommodate the controlling area.

8) In order to be able to coordinate and tolerate the changes, both areas will need to be addressed in the session or lesson. In fact, many times one needs to include attention to all the joints, to negotiate specific or significant changes elsewhere in the body.

I encourage you to explore the above ideas, to take your seeing skills into problem solving your session design and to be most helpful to your clients interests and limitations.

We have covered a lot of information.
Upon coming to this book, many of you had already acquired great skill in seeing body alignment in relation to the plumb line. Perhaps now you can widen your focus to appreciate more of the information the body offers, by observing dimension, force of gravity and GRF, asymmetry, range of neutral, alignment, and function.

In actuality, every body has its current best available neutral and its own emerging model. Rather than prescribing a postural model, I trust that you now understand the information in this book is to be used as a guideline – a reference to expand your current understanding and another starting point for study. It is also an invitation to explore the many applications of these ideas about posture, movement and expression. I hope you will use whatever sections of this book best meet your interests and needs.

Judith Aston
2019

TO CONTACT US

How these seeing and evaluation skills are applied to the other Aston forms of movement (Aston-Kinetics), bodywork (Aston-Massage, Arthro-Kinetics and Myo-Kinetics), ergonomics and fitness, is beyond the scope of this manual. If you are interested in furthering your exploration of the Aston Paradigm and techniques, please visit our website at AstonKinetics.com or send us a message at office@astonkinetics.com, to be put on our mailing list for classes, events and products.